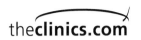
theclinics.com

ANESTHESIOLOGY CLINICS

New Vistas in Patient Safety and Simulation

GUEST EDITORS
W. Andrew Kofke, MD,
and Vinay M. Nadkarni, MD

CONSULTING EDITOR
Lee A. Fleisher, MD

June 2007 • Volume 25 • Number 2

SAUNDERS

An Imprint of Elsevier, Inc.
PHILADELPHIA   LONDON   TORONTO   MONTREAL   SYDNEY   TOKYO

W.B. SAUNDERS COMPANY
A Division of Elsevier Inc.

1600 John F. Kennedy Boulevard, Suite 1800 • Philadelphia, Pennsylvania 19103-2899

http://www.theclinics.com

ANESTHESIOLOGY CLINICS   Volume 25, Number 2
June 2007   ISSN 1932-2275
Editor: Rachel Glover   ISBN-13: 978-1-4160-4279-2
                                                                    ISBN-10: 1-4160-4279-2

The ideas and opinions expressed in *Anesthesiology Clinics* do not necessarily reflect those of the Publisher. The Publisher does not assume any responsibility for any injury and/or damage to persons or property arising out of or related to any use of the material contained in this periodical. The reader is advised to check the appropriate medical literature and the product information currently provided by the manufacturer of each drug to be administered to verify the dosage, the method and duration of administration, or contraindications. It is the responsibility of the treating physician or other health care professional, relying on independent experience and knowledge of the patient, to determine drug dosages and the best treatment for the patient. Mention of any product in this issue should not be construed as endorsement by the contributors, editors, or the Publisher of the product or manufacturers' claims.

Anesthesiology Clinics (ISSN 1932-2275) is published quarterly by Elsevier Inc., 360 Park Avenue South, New York, NY 10010-1710. Months of issue are March, June, September, and December. Business and Editorial Offices: 1600 John F. Kennedy Blvd., Suite 1800, Philadelphia, PA 19103-2899. Customer Service Office: 6277 Sea Harbor Drive, Orlando, FL 32887-4800. Periodicals postage paid at New York, NY and additional mailing offices. Subscription prices are $101.00 per year (US student/resident), $202.00 per year (US individuals), $246.00 per year (Canadian individuals), $302.00 per year (US institutions), $366.00 per year (Canadian institutions), $134.00 per year (Canadian and foreign student/resident), $263.00 per year (foreign individuals), and $366.00 per year (foreign institutions). To receive student and resident rate, orders must be accompanied by name of affiliated institution, date of term, and the *signature* of program/residency coordinator on institutions letterhead. Orders will be billed at individual rate until proof of status is received. Foreign air speed delivery is included in all *Clinics'* subscription prices. All prices are subject to change without notice. POSTMASTER: Send address changes to *Anesthesiology Clinics*, Elsevier Periodicals Customer Service, 6277 Sea Harbor Drive, Orlando, FL 32887-4800. **Customer Service: 1-800-654-2452** (US). From outside of the US, call **1-407-345-4000**. E-mail: hhspcs@wbsaunders.com.

Anesthesiology Clinics, is also published in Spanish by McGraw-Hill Inter-americana Editores S. A., P.O. Box 5-237, 06500 Mexico D. F., Mexico.

Anesthesiology Clinics, is covered in *Index Medicus, Current Contents/Clinical Medicine, Excerpta Medica, ISI/BIOMED,* and *Chemical Abstracts.*

Printed in the United States of America.

CONSULTING EDITOR

LEE A. FLEISHER, MD, Robert D. Dripps Professor of Medicine; Chair, Anesthesiology and Critical Care, The University of Pennsylvania School of Medicine, Philadelphia, Pennsylvania

GUEST EDITORS

W. ANDREW KOFKE, MD, Professor and Director, Neuroanesthesia; Co-director, Neurocritical Care; Medical Director, Measey Simulation Center of the School of Medicine, Departments of Anesthesia and Neurosurgery, University of Pennsylvania, Philadelphia, Pennsylvania

VINAY M. NADKARNI, MD, Division of Critical Care, Department of Anesthesiology and Critical Care Medicine, The Children's Hospital of Philadelphia, Philadelphia; Department of Anesthesiology and Critical Care, University of Pennsylvania School of Medicine, Philadelphia, Pennsylvania

CONTRIBUTORS

P. PAT BANERJEE, PhD, Professor, Department of Mechanical and Industrial Engineering, Computer Science, Bioengineering, University of Illinois–Chicago, Chicago, Illinois

HAIM BERKENSTADT, MD, Deputy Director, The Israel Center for Medical Simulation (MSR), Sheba Medical Center, Tel-Hashomer; Tel Aviv University Sackler School of Medicine, Jerusalem; The Israeli Board Examination Committee in Anesthesiology, Jerusalem, Israel

RICHARD BLUM, MD, Assistant Professor, Anesthesiology, Harvard Medical School, Children's Hospital, Boston, Massachusetts

MARY J. CANTRELL, MA, Director, Center for Clinical Skills Education and Standardized Patient Program, University of Arkansas for Medical Sciences, Little Rock; Director, PULSE Center, Arkansas Children's Hospital, Arkansas

LINDA A. DELONEY, EdD, Medical Educator, Department of Radiology, College of Medicine, University of Arkansas for Medical Sciences, Little Rock, Arkansas

PARVATI DEV, PhD, Director, SUMMIT, Stanford University School of Medicine, Stanford, California

DAWN DILLMAN, MD, Associate Professor of Anesthesiology and Perioperative Medicine, Department of Anesthesiology and Perioperative Medicine, Oregon Health and Science University, Portland, Oregon

RONALD L. DUFRESNE, PhD, Assistant Professor, Department of Management, Haub School of Business, Saint Joseph's University, Philadelphia, Pennsylvania

DAVID FARRIS, MD, Private Practitioner, Chief of CV Anesthesia, Medical Director, Bloodless Medicine Program, Legacy Emanuel Hospital, Legacy Health System, Portland; and Emanuel Children's Hospital, Portland, Oregon

DAVID FEINSTEIN, MD, Assistant Professor, Anesthesiology, Harvard Medical School, Beth Israel Deaconess Medical Center, Boston, Massachusetts

CRAIG GLAIBERMAN, MD, Assistant Professor, Radiology, Mallinckrodt Institute of Radiology, Washington University School of Medicine, St Louis, Missouri

DEREK A. GOULD, MBChB, FRCP, FRCR, Consultant Interventional Radiologist; Honorary Reader, Royal Liverpool University Hospital, Prescot Street, Liverpool, United Kingdom

W. LEROY HEINRICHS, MD, PhD, Associate Director, SUMMIT, Stanford University School of Medicine, Stanford, California

ELIZABETH A. HUNT, MD, MPH, Director, Johns Hopkins Simulation Center; Assistant Professor, Department of Anesthesiology and Critical Care Medicine, Johns Hopkins University School of Medicine, Baltimore, Maryland

RON KEREN, MD, MPH, Division of General Pediatrics, The Children's Hospital of Philadelphia; Department of Pediatrics, University of Pennsylvania School of Medicine, Philadelphia, Pennsylvania

CRISTIAN J. LUCIANO, MS, Research Assistant, Department of Mechanical and Industrial Engineering, University of Illinois-Chicago, Chicago, Illinois

LAURA KUSUMOTO, PhD, Vice President, Forterra Studios, Forterra Systems, San Mateo, California

VINAY M. NADKARNI, MD, Division of Critical Care, Department of Anesthesiology and Critical Care Medicine, The Children's Hospital of Philadelphia, Philadelphia; Department of Anesthesiology and Critical Care, University of Pennsylvania School of Medicine, Philadelphia, Pennsylvania

KRISTEN L. NELSON, MD, Pediatric Critical Care Fellow, Johns Hopkins Simulation Center, Department of Anesthesiology and Critical Care Medicine, Johns Hopkins University School of Medicine, Baltimore, Maryland

AKIRA NISHISAKI, MD, Division of Critical Care, Department of Anesthesiology and Critical Care Medicine, The Children's Hospital of Philadelphia, Philadelphia; Division of General Pediatrics, The Children's Hospital of Philadelphia, Philadelphia, Pennsylvania

AALPEN A. PATEL, MD, Assistant Professor of Radiology (and Surgery), Department of Radiology, University of Pennsylvania School of Medicine, Hospital of the University of Pennsylvania, Philadelphia, Pennsylvania

JOHN PAWLOWSKI, MD, PhD, Assistant Professor, Anesthesiology, Harvard Medical School, Beth Israel Deaconess Medical Center, Boston, Massachusetts

STEPHEN PRATT, MD, Assistant Professor, Anesthesiology, Harvard Medical School, Beth Israel Deaconess Medical Center, Boston, Massachusetts

DANIEL B. RAEMER, PhD, Program Director, Center for Medical Simulation, Cambridge; Associate Professor in Anesthesia, Harvard Medical School and Massachusetts General Hospital, Boston, Massachusetts

PETER RIVARD, PhD, Postdoctoral Fellow, Center for Organization, Leadership and Management Research, VA Boston Healthcare System, Boston, Massachusetts

SILVIO RIZZI, MS, Research Assistant, Department of Mechanical and Industrial Engineering, University of Illinois–Chicago, Chicago, Illinois

ORIT RUBIN, PhD, The Israel Center for Medical Simulation (MSR), Sheba Medical Center, Tel-Hashomer; The National Institute for Testing and Evaluation, Jerusalem, Israel

JENNY W. RUDOLPH, PhD, Assistant Professor, Department of Health Policy and Management, Boston University School of Public Health, Boston; Center for Medical Simulation, Cambridge, Massachusetts

MICHAEL SEROPIAN, MD, FRCPC, Associate Professor of Anesthesiology and Perioperative Medicine, Department of Anesthesiology and Perioperative Medicine, Oregon Health and Science University, Portland, Oregon; Founder and Past Director, OHSU Simulation Center, Portland, Oregon; Member, Board of Directors, Society for Simulation in Healthcare; Chair-Elect, Oregon Simulation Alliance

NICOLE A. SHILKOFSKI, MD, Pediatric Critical Care Fellow, Johns Hopkins Simulation Center, Department of Anesthesiology and Critical Care Medicine, Johns Hopkins University School of Medicine, Baltimore, Maryland

AVNER SIDI, MD, Tel Aviv University Sackler School of Medicine, Jerusalem; The Israeli Board Examination Committee in Anesthesiology, Jerusalem; Vice Chairman, Department of Anesthesiology and Intensive Care, Sheba Medical Center, Tel-Hashomer, Israel

ROBERT SIMON, EdD, Education Director, Center for Medical Simulation, Cambridge; Instructor in Anesthesia, Harvard Medical School and Massachusetts General Hospital, Boston, Massachusetts

ELIZABETH H. SINZ, MD, Associate Professor, Departments of Anesthesiology and Neurosurgery; Director, Simulation Development and Cognitive Science Laboratory, Pennsylvania State University College of Medicine, Penn State Hershey Medical Center, Hershey, Pennsylvania

STEPHEN D. SMALL, MD, Assistant Professor, Department of Anesthesiology and Critical Care, University of Chicago, Chicago; Director, Center for Simulation and Safety in Healthcare, University of Chicago, Chicago, Illinois

THEODORA A. STAVROUDIS, MD, Neonatology Fellow, Johns Hopkins Simulation Center, Department of Pediatrics, Johns Hopkins University School of Medicine, Baltimore, Maryland

ESWAR SUNDAR, MD, Instructor, Anesthesiology, Harvard Medical School, Beth Israel Deaconess Medical Center, Boston, Massachusetts

SUGANTHA SUNDAR, MD, Instructor, Anesthesiology, Harvard Medical School, Beth Israel Deaconess Medical Center, Boston, Massachusetts

PATRICIA YOUNGBLOOD, PhD, Director of Evaluation, SUMMIT, Stanford University School of Medicine, Stanford, California

AMITAI ZIV, MD, MHA, Director, The Israel Center for Medical Simulation (MSR), Sheba Medical Center, Tel-Hashomer; Tel Aviv University Sackler School of Medicine, Jerusalem, Israel

CONTENTS

performance in clinical settings. However, no evidence yet shows that crew resource management training through simulation, despite its promise, improves team operational performance at the bedside. Also, no evidence to date proves that simulation training actually improves patient outcome. Even so, confidence is growing in the validity of medical simulation as the training tool of the future. The use of medical simulation will continue to grow in the context of multidisciplinary team training for patient safety.

Simulation applications have become increasingly common in health care. A convergence of factors has stimulated this growth, including the rapid advance of enabling technologies, demand for improved outcomes and objectively assessed competencies, and translation of lessons learned from other high-risk industries as a function of the patient safety and quality movements. The bulk of the experience gained and resources expended has been focused on education, training, and assessment of clinicians' knowledge, skills, and attitudes. Simulation methods lend themselves to supporting human factors and systems-level investigations, yet work in health care has, to a large degree, been limited to a few experienced centers, interdisciplinary research teams, and isolated novel studies.

Assessment and evaluation are integral parts of any educational and training process, and students at all levels of training respond by studying more seriously for the parts of the course or training that are assessed. To promote and enhance effective learning successfully, simulation and other teaching methods should be both formative and summative, because the ultimate goal is to ensure professional competence. This article describes a model of medical competence, and focuses on the use of medical simulation in assessment and evaluation of different levels of clinical competence using examples from experience.

Statewide simulation networks afford not only the possibility of meeting capacity needs for anesthesiologists, but also provide a venue for training trainers, setting standards, and bringing academic and nonacademic practices together. Furthermore, a statewide network that is appropriately designed opens the door to interdisciplinary activity. Oregon is the first state to implement simulation education across disciplines throughout the state. The model provides an example of how simulation can be successfully applied across a large and diverse area. The article details the benefits of statewide simulation networks, discusses challenges to implementing such networks, and describes Oregon's statewide efforts.

This article reviews medical team training using the principles of crew resource management (CRM). It also briefly discusses crisis resource management, a subset of CRM, as applied to high-acuity medical situations. Guidelines on setting up medical team training programs are presented. Team training programs are classified and examples of simulation-based and classroom-based programs are offered and their merits discussed. Finally, a brief look at the future of team training concludes this review article.

Traditional medical education has emphasized autonomy, and until recently issues related to teamwork have not been explicitly included in medical curriculum. The Institute of Medicine highlighted that health care providers train as individuals, yet function as teams, creating a gap between training and reality and called for the use of medical simulation to improve teamwork. The aviation industry created a program called Cockpit and later Crew Resource Management that has served as a model for team training programs in medicine. This article reviews important concepts related to teamwork and discusses examples where simulation either could be or has been used to improve teamwork in medical disciplines to enhance patient safety.

An important component of all emergency medicine residency programs is managing trauma effectively as a member of an emergency medicine team, but practice on live patients is often impractical and mannequin-based simulators are expensive and require all trainees to be physically present at the same location. This article describes a project to develop and evaluate a computer-based simulator (the Virtual Emergency Department) for distance training in teamwork and leadership in trauma management. The virtual environment provides repeated practice opportunities with life-threatening trauma cases in a safe and reproducible setting.

FORTHCOMING ISSUES

RECENT ISSUES

ANESTHESIOLOGY
CLINICS

Anesthesiology Clin
25 (2007) xiii–xiv

Foreword

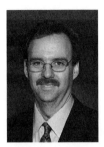

Lee A. Fleisher, MD
Consulting Editor

Anesthesiology has been praised among all medical specialties for embracing patient safety and implementing changes leading to best outcomes. For the most part, these advances have been the result of using technology and developing standards and guidelines for care. Despite the accolades the specialty has received, individuals in the specialty have continued to innovate in this area, particularly beyond the initial goals of teaching clinical skills. In this issue of Clinics, the editors have taken a comprehensive look at how simulation can be used in diverse ways, including the important concept of team training.

As guest editors for this issue, we are fortunate to have W. Andrew Kofke, MD, and Vinay Nadkarni, MD. Dr Kofke is Professor of Anesthesiology at the University of Pennsylvania School of Medicine and an attending anesthesiologist at the Hospital of the University of Pennsylvania. He is Director of Neuroanesthesia and Director of the Measy Simulation Center of the University of Pennsylvania and has been involved in simulation at the University of Pittsburgh and West Virginia University. Dr Nadkarni is Associate Professor of Anesthesiology and Critical Care and Pediatrics at the University of Pennsylvania and an attending pediatric intensivist at the Children's Hospital of Philadelphia. He is a recognized expert in pediatric

doi:10.1016/j.anclin.2007.04.002   *anesthesiology.theclinics.com*

resuscitation. Together they are in an excellent position to provide readers with comprehensive information about the use of simulation from world-renowned experts.

Lee A. Fleisher, MD
Anesthesiology and Critical Care
University of Pennsylvania
6 Dulles, 3400 Spruce Street
Philadelphia, PA 19104, USA

E-mail address: fleishel@uphs.upenn.edu

ELSEVIER
SAUNDERS

Anesthesiology Clin
25 (2007) xv–xix

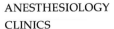

ANESTHESIOLOGY
CLINICS

Preface

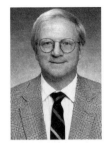 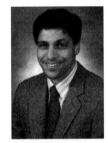

W. Andrew Kofke, MD   Vinay M. Nadkarni, MD
Guest Editors

December 7, 1941, Pearl Harbor. Lots of casualties. Routine patient safety efforts primarily consist of finger on the pulse, eyes on the chest, observation of skin color. The recently released drug, thiopental, is employed. Some of the soldiers die...of anesthesia [1–3]. Anesthesia-related death rate reported at one in 450 [2].

September 1979—September 1981. Anesthesiology residency. The operating surgeon calmly says, "Blood's dark." The resident's reaction: BLOOD'S DARK!!! The alarmed resident recollects in a moment the repeated lessons of an instructor: The first three things to check for with any problem in the operating room are first airway, then the airway, and finally the airway. So the resident checks the airway and finds a disconnect that somehow was not heard with the esophageal stethoscope over the orthopedists' hammers and drills. No oxygen analyzer, no disconnect alarm, no pulse oximeter, no automated blood pressure monitor; by today's standards, no nothing, although anesthesiologists did have manual blood pressure cuffs, EKG machines, and the beginnings of advanced hemodynamic monitoring. The resident's attendings were fond of saying, "When I was a resident..." followed by some parable of how he managed with no monitors other than his five senses. It seemed like at least once a year at morbidity and mortality (M&M) there was discussion about an intraoperative death by undetected disconnect. Anesthesia death rate said to be about one in 10,000.

2007. Cyanosis is virtually never seen by trainees and death by disconnect is now unheard of. Gas analyzers, pulse oximetry, end-tidal carbon dioxide, easily balanced pressure monitors, idiot-proof machines, and more are part

1932-2275/07/$ - see front matter © 2007 Elsevier Inc. All rights reserved.
doi:10.1016/j.anclin.2007.04.001   *anesthesiology.theclinics.com*

of the modern anesthesia toolbox. Anesthesia death rate in healthy patients thought to be about one in 200,000 [4,5]. Remarkable progress.

The Anesthesia Patient Safety Foundation (APSF) was formed September 30, 1985, by Ellison Pierce with the help of many others. The efforts of the APSF (http://www.apsf.org/) have produced in the patient care environment this remarkable transformation, which arose initially in the operating room, and now is spreading to general medical, surgical, and pediatric floors; emergency departments; and intensive care units. The accomplishments of the specialty of anesthesiology in advancing patient safety have been so successful that they have been emulated by other medical specialties and the patient safety movement has morphed into the multidisciplinary National Patient Safety Foundation (http://www.npsf.org/), which will undoubtedly address many of the patient safety issues outside of operating rooms now recognized as widespread. Indeed, the notion of patient safety started by these visionaries has now infected the culture of medicine and it is now the buzzword of quality improvement programs everywhere. However, a problem remains among health care practitioners following the "watch one, do one, teach one" mantra from the Flexner era and before, leading current visionaries to conceive and promulgate simulation as an educational tool to advance patient safety.

Simulation, as defined by the Center for Medical Simulation, Cambridge, Massachusetts, is a situation or environment created to allow persons to experience a representation of a real event for the purpose of practicing, learning, evaluating, or testing, or to gain understanding of systems or human actions.

Back in 1967, Red Cross first aid classes taught a recently described resuscitation method called cardiopulmonary resuscitation (CPR). CPR took the place of the chest-pressure–arm-lift method, the primary resuscitation method of the 1950s and 1960s and perhaps before. So what did we practice our CPR on? Resusci Anne. At that time, Resusci Anne was a new Laerdal product used everywhere to teach mouth-to-mouth resuscitation and chest compressions following the contemporary recommendations of the American Heart Association. By today's standards, this was a primitive simulator. It is, however, still in use.

A far more sophisticated simulator, perhaps the most sophisticated simulator ever made, was Sim One, demonstrated in the late 1960s by Stephen Abrahamson, founding chair of the Department of Education at the University of Southern California [6]. He and his coworkers developed the high-fidelity simulator; which is more sophisticated than the simulators currently available. Sim One even fasciculated after injection of succinylcholine. However, it required a roomful of computers, each with an attendant technician in the manner of a NASA space launch. Dr Abrahamson went on sabbatical, his simulator was dismantled, so the story goes, and it took advances in computer technology and the vision of subsequent simulation pioneers to resurrect this technology in the 1990s. The field of simulation is now growing exponentially. In the early 1990s, the number of simulation centers was less than 100. Now, in 2007, over 1,000 simulation centers operate worldwide.

The taxonomy of simulation can be characterized as follows:

- **Task training**. The use of simulation devices intended to teach specific psychomotor tasks with complexity ranging from simple insertion of an intravenous cannula into a simulated arm to a computerized virtual reality world that allows an operator to learn highly complex surgical procedures, such as laparoscopy or endoscopy procedures. These topics will be reviewed in several articles in this issue.
- **Personal-computer–based simulation**. The use of personal-computer–based programs installed on laptop computers. They can be set up to mimic real-life scenarios such that the user has to encounter the important spectrum of cognitive decision algorithms required in clinical practice. Moreover, in accord with evolving preferences of younger generations, the computer-based simulation can also be set up as a game.
- **Standardized patients**. What can be better than working on a real human? This notion has resulted in the development of standardized patient programs in many schools and a standardized patient society (www.aspeducators.org), the subject of Mary Cantrell's article in this issue. Standardized patients are real people. That is, they are individuals trained to display the appropriate behaviors of patients with given diseases in given situations or they are individuals with the relevant physical findings. Both types of standardized patients can be used to teach novices how to deal with a variety of problems. Good examples of such standardized patients are women who volunteer to undergo pelvic examinations by medical students. These women use their acting skills to feign a patient's symptom and behavior complex, and then provide constructive feedback to the students.
- **High-fidelity simulation**. This uses simulators that bring together all of the physiologic and pharmacologic responses of a human in a manikin that breathes, may produce or consume a variety of different gases, and talks in an interactive manner with students. After appropriate suspension of disbelief, this manikin becomes for all intents and purposes a real human being with a real problem that students have to diagnose and treat appropriately.

All of these elements of simulation can be further integrated to create scenarios encompassing any or all of these methods. Students can perform procedures, make decisions, and interact with a patient (manikin or standardized patient), which may be attached to a task trainer. At an even higher level, students may interact with other health care providers on a team. Team training and performance can be taught, learned, performed, and practiced. This has led to the increasing use of such simulation tools to train health care providers in the principles of crew or crisis resource management (teamwork), a lesson from the aviation industry, also reviewed in articles in this issue. Finally, simulation can be used as an essential tool for micro- or macro-system simulations. Such simulations help students learn how to handle multiple patients and manage multiple medical, interpersonal, and system issues. The use of simulations in such applications also is reviewed in this issue.

Simulation is increasingly used to improve the self-confidence, competence, and operational performance of health care providers, which ultimately improves patient safety and patient outcomes. In summary, we have made significant progress in patient safety, but there remains a need for practitioners to use methods found to be helpful in high-reliability organizations, such as the airline and nuclear energy industries. Based on these organizations' excellent safety records, it becomes logical to suggest that simulations of rare events, for experienced practitioners, and common events, for the inexperienced practitioner, should be the next vista in patient safety. The various contributions to this issue make it clear that many advances are emerging in this field and that the medical culture of this century is going to be extraordinarily different from that of the last. We are going to transition from "see one, do one, teach one," to a culture of "practice it 'til proficient and then, and only then, do one." Indeed, we should not be surprised to find in the twenty-first century the routine use of high-stakes simulation for certification and hospital credentialing. These advances represent an important cultural shift in medicine, a shift that is still evolving and that will include many of the new vistas glimpsed in this issue.

W. Andrew Kofke, MD
University of Pennsylvania
7 Dulles Bldg.
3400 Spruce St.
Philadelphia, PA 19104, USA

E-mail address: Andrew.Kofke@uphs.upenn.edu

Vinay M. Nadkarni, MD
Division of Critical Care
Department of Anesthesiology and Critical Care Medicine
The Children's Hospital of Philadelphia
34th St. and Civic Center Blvd.
Philadelphia, PA 19104, USA

Department of Anesthesiology and Critical Care
University of Pennsylvania School of Medicine
Philadelphia, PA 19104, USA

E-mail address: nadkarni@email.chop.edu

References

[1] Moorhead JJ. Surgical experience at Pearl Harbor. J Am Med Assoc 1942;118:712–4.
[2] Beecher HK. Anesthesia for men wounded in battle. In: Coates JB, De Bakey MF. editors. Surgery in World War II medical department United States army 1955;2:70–4.
[3] Bennetts FE. Thiopentone anaesthesia at Pearl Harbor. Br J Anaesth 1995;75:366–8.
[4] Eichhorn JH. Prevention of intraoperative anesthesia accidents and related severe injury through safety monitoring. Anesthesiology 1989;70:572–7.
[5] Lagasse RS. Anesthesia safety: model or myth? Anesthesiology 2002;97:1609–17.
[6] Guilbert JJ. Making a difference: an interview of Professor Stephen Abrahamson. Education for Health 2003;16(3):378–84.

ANESTHESIOLOGY
CLINICS

Anesthesiology Clin
25 (2007) 209–223

Anesthesiology National CME Program and ASA Activities in Simulation

Elizabeth H. Sinz, MD

Departments of Anesthesiology and Neurosurgery, Simulation Development and Cognitive Science Laboratory, Office of Education Affairs, Pennsylvania State University College of Medicine, Penn State Hershey Medical Center, H187, 500 University Drive, P.O. Box 850, Hershey, PA 17033-0850, USA

Simulation-based teaching has been used for health care training for many decades. Yet, only in the past few years has interest in this modality exploded. Historically, anesthesiology has been at the forefront of full-scale patient simulation. Now, all disciplines of health care education have embraced simulation-based learning. Why all of the interest in simulation now? Where do anesthesiologists stand on the issue of simulation-based teaching? How is the American Society of Anesthesiologists (ASA) involved? This article explores the history of anesthesiology's role in simulation and the latest endeavors of the ASA to promote simulation-based instruction.

For many years, anesthesiologists have used simulation models for practice and training in resuscitation. In the 1950s, Peter Safar paralyzed human volunteers and showed they could be kept oxygenated and ventilated using the new mouth-to-mouth technique (Fig. 1) [1]. Safar and Bjørn Lind, both anesthesiologists, worked with Åsmund S. Lærdal, a toy manufacturer with extensive experience and knowledge of plastics, to build a life-sized "doll" for teaching and practicing the new resuscitation technique of mouth-to-mouth ventilation [2,3]. Because of its simplicity and portability, this early simulator, the Resusci Anne, continues to be used after more than four decades to train basic life-support skills.

With the advent of the computer age, a truly amazing invention, the Sim One Anesthesiological Simulator, was conceived and built by medical educator Stephen Abrahamson and anesthesiologist J. Samuel Denson at the University of Southern California in Los Angeles with a group of engineers

E-mail address: esinz@psu.edu

doi:10.1016/j.anclin.2007.03.012 *anesthesiology.theclinics.com*

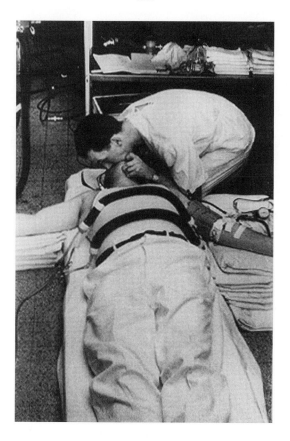

**BALTIMORE CITY HOSPITAL
RESUSCITATION EXPERIMENT, JULY 13, 1957
CHEST PRESSURE ARM-LIFT METHOD**

Fig. 1. Peter Safar performing mouth-to-mouth ventilation on a chemically paralyzed volunteer. (*Courtesy of* Safar Center for Resuscitation Research, Pitts burgh, PA; with permission. Copyright © 1998–2002, Safar Center for Resuscitation Research. All rights reserved worldwide.)

from Aerojet-General Corporation. This prototype device, which required a separate room for the attached computer, was never copied but was used with success for airway training and anesthesiology-events teaching in the late 1960s and early 1970s (Fig. 2) [4–9]. In the early 1980s while performing animal experiments related to cardiopulmonary bypasses, another anesthesiologist, David Gaba, began to consider decision-making during patient emergencies. By then, Sim One was long gone. So, rather than have health care teams practice on animals, Gaba and his colleagues developed a new artificial human. By 1986, advanced computer technology, engineering, and plastics had been incorporated into the Virtual Anesthesiology

July 14, 1970   S. ABRAHAMSON ET AL   3,520,071

ANESTHESIOLOGICAL TRAINING SIMULATOR

Filed Jan. 29, 1968   11 Sheets–Sheet 1

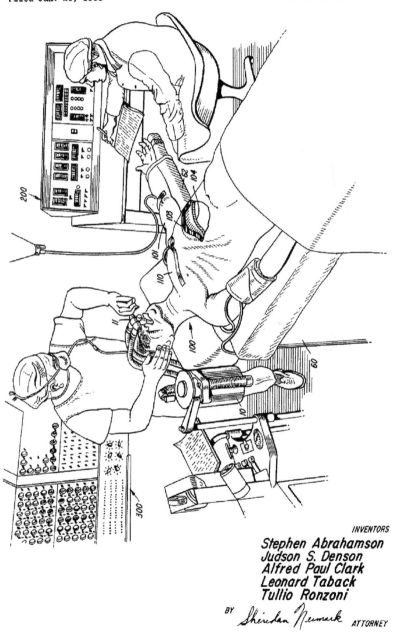

INVENTORS
Stephen Abrahamson
Judson S. Denson
Alfred Paul Clark
Leonard Taback
Tullio Ronzoni

BY *Sheridan Neumark* ATTORNEY

Fig. 2. Patent application for Sim One. (*From* Abrahamson S, Denson JS, Clark AP, et al. Anesthesiological training simulator. US Patent Office, Patent No. 3,520,071, July 14, 1970.)

Training Simulation System, which provided a realistic way to practice patient emergencies [10,11]. Crew resource management, a planned approach to team training from the airline industry, was adapted and initially called anesthesia crisis resource management [12–14].

Howard Schwid [15,16] developed interactive flat-screen anesthesiology computer simulations that allowed individuals to manage a wide variety of complicated cases and patient complications using readily available computers. This easier, cheaper approach, though less realistic than a full-scale patient simulation, does not require an on-site instructor, which is needed with a full-scale patient simulation. Anesthesia simulator development has generally paralleled advances in technology, especially computer technology.

The inherently dangerous nature of anesthesia drove the development of simulation applications for anesthesiology, which began to address patient safety in a scientific, proactive manner in the late 1970s. The ASA undertook a massive effort to reduce anesthetic-related morbidity and mortality first by focusing on finding ways to avoid the causes of anesthetic-related morbidity and mortality [17]. In 1985, the Anesthesia Patient Safety Foundation (APSF) was created to focus on patient safety, and some of Gaba's early simulation work was funded by an APSF grant [18,19]. In 1986, the ASA was the first medical specialty society to adopt standards of care for its members (http://www.apsf.org/).

Throughout the 1990s, the field of anesthesiology continued to improve patient safety and many educators began to use simulation to improve safety in the operating room. Full-scale human patient simulation was favored for practicing team skills and responses to rare clinical events. Procedural skills formerly practiced mostly on animals or people were increasingly practiced using "task trainers" that felt increasingly realistic as materials and anatomic models improved. Virtual reality devices incorporated haptic modeling to provide realistic response and sense of touch based on the actions of the trainee. Other specialties began to study simulation-based teaching. It became apparent that the initial learning curve for many procedures can be shortened through the use of virtual reality simulation training [20–26], confirming the impressions from the early days of Sim One [7].

The use of simulation is now advocated when introducing new products and techniques to otherwise fully trained, practicing physicians. Currently one product, the Cordis Angioguard, a carotid stent from Johnson & Johnson, carries a recommendation from the US Food and Drug Administration that practitioners demonstrate proficiency in its placement on a simulator before using the device on patients [27]. This type of credentialing may become commonplace for new products [28]. Many advocates of simulation have focused on procedural training because of the relative ease of measuring outcomes with and without simulation-based practice. Surprisingly, physicians have never before been required to formally demonstrate competence with a procedure before performing it on patients.

Meanwhile, changing attitudes among patients and educators progressively made it more difficult, especially for beginners, to practice key skills on real people. Changes in reimbursement requirements have made it difficult for medical students to gain practical experience in patient care while under the careful watch of teaching physicians. The privacy rules included in the Health Insurance Portability and Accountability Act have sometimes been invoked to discourage medical students from even observing patient care or reviewing real cases. The decrease in actual patient care during medical school has pushed the burden of practical training into residency. However, concurrent changes in resident work hours and a real reduction in reimbursement for clinical teaching have also reduced the ability of residents to gain adequate practical experience during residency. One potential solution to the reduced time for clinical practice might be a longer residency. However, this is practically impossible because of the incredible debt carried by many upon graduation from medical school. The competing demands of patient safety versus the need for rigorous physician education have inevitably led to proposals that simulation-based training might solve inherent flaws in the current education system [29,30].

ASA workgroup on simulation education headed by Michael A. Olympio

Simulation became a regular topic at meetings of the Society for Education in Anesthesia (SEA) and the Society for Technology in Anesthesia (STA) by the late 1990s. In 2002, at a meeting in Orlando Florida, the ASA held its first full-scale simulation-based workshop. In 2004, the ASA formally began the process of delineating opportunities for anesthesiologists to obtain quality continuing medical education (CME) credit in a simulation-based environment by creating an ad-hoc Workgroup on Simulation Education, which was chaired by Michael Olympio (Table 1). This workgroup met repeatedly over a 2-year span and developed a white paper (available at http://www.asahq.org/SIM/ASASimWhitePaper071806.pdf) that outlines the rationale and plan, endorsed by the ASA, for implementation of simulation-based CME for anesthesiologists.

The workgroup began by conducting a survey to gauge the attitudes and concerns of ASA members regarding simulation-based CME opportunities [31]. This poll, placed on the ASA Web site, generated responses from 1,350 ASA members with 80% indicating they were interested in simulation-based CME and only 9% saying they were uncomfortable or not interested in this type of learning. Most respondents (88%) indicated that convenient course locations would be an important drawing factor, so decentralization was deemed an important characteristic. In addition, 90% of those polled wanted simulation experiences to improve their management of rare or difficult events and 79% wanted to practice crisis resource management or teamwork. Because of the poll's methodology, those who responded were

Table 1
Members of the ASA Workgroup on Simulation Education

Name	Affiliation
Anita Abbatacola	American Society of Anesthesiologists
Paul Barach	University of Miami
Ellen Bateman	American Society of Anesthesiologists
Dan Cole	The Mayo Clinic
Jeff Cooper	Massachusetts General Hospital, Harvard Medical
David Gaba	Stanford University
Glenn Gravlee	The Ohio State University
Adam Levine	New York University
Gary Loyd	West Virginia University
Michael Olympio	Wake Forest University
Janice Plack	American Society of Anesthesiologists
Joseph Quinlan	University of Pittsburgh
Keith Ruskin	Yale University
John Schaefer	Medical University of South Carolina
Michael Seropian	Oregon Health Sciences University
Elizabeth Sinz	Pennsylvania State University
Randolph Steadman	University of California at Los Angeles
Jeff Taekman	Duke University
Laurence Torsher	The Mayo Clinic
Matthew Weinger	Vanderbilt University
David Wilks	University of New Mexico

probably more interested than the general membership in simulation-based learning. Even so, the strong support for simulation coupled with the growing use of simulation-based teaching in residency training programs and at ASA and component society meetings encouraged the workgroup to press ahead.

The poll also identified several important barriers to participation in simulation-based CME. Several individuals commented on the poor fidelity of currently available simulators, an issue that becomes more relevant and problematic with more experienced clinicians. There was also a concern that participants could feel intimidated or be embarrassed, particularly when recordings and group sessions are used for teaching. The increased cost associated with simulation-based teaching, compared with lectures, was also deemed a barrier, and the workgroup considered the possibility of increased CME credit for time spent in simulation-based education. Respondents also expressed a variety of concerns related to the use of simulation-based testing or credentialing and questioned whether the current models were adequate for high-stakes assessment. The workgroup was mindful of these concerns throughout the development of the white paper, which provides a course of action that will foster and delineate worthwhile simulation-based CME opportunities for ASA members.

The workgroup also developed a Web-based registry of simulation centers interested in providing simulation-based CME (available at http://simulation.asahq.org/search/index.asp.) As of the end of 2006, there were 31 simulation centers listed with short descriptions of each center and Web site links. This Web-based resource will eventually list all ASA-approved programs and courses, and will inform the ASA membership about each program's status in the ASA approval process. ASA members will have this resource for locating endorsed simulation-based educational opportunities. In addition, the registry will provide simulation programs with a means of advertising their CME programs, thus providing ASA support for the programs.

The workgroup developed a common language to describe the various components of a simulation program, creating several new terms in the process (Appendix 1). Essential elements of every simulation program include (1) a program director, (2) simulation instructors, (3) content experts, (4) courses, and (5) course directors. There are currently no generally accepted systems for credentialing or certifying any of these elements. The workgroup developed a template for simulation program approval criteria that allows flexibility for providing evidence for the high level of educational value desired by ASA members.

Programs may exist within a simulation center, or they may be independently operated, but they are defined by the courses that are offered. Each program must have a program director with the authority to lead a simulation program by virtue of his or her knowledge of simulation-based instruction and his or her ability to organize courses. Each course must also have a course director who is a current member of the ASA. However, additional instructors knowledgeable about the specific educational content may also be employed. Every course must also involve a certified simulation instructor who is knowledgeable about simulation-based educational techniques. One ASA member with credentials could serve as both a simulation instructor and a content expert. Because there is currently no standard process for becoming a simulation education expert, the process for becoming a certified simulation instructor relies on a portfolio summarizing that individual's credentials and experience. Assessment of these portfolios must rely on reviews by a subcommittee using a semi-objective approach. In the future, specific coursework may be required for instructors. Currently, several good courses are offered by different institutions to introduce and practice simulation-based teaching skills. Content experts can be chosen by the program director, but experts will generally be expected to hold a doctoral-level degree in their areas of expertise.

Nine basic criteria were identified for ASA program approval (Appendix 2). These criteria are intended to not only provide the minimal requirements for program approval, but also to encourage continual improvements in programs, centers, and instructors. Review by the ASA is essential, but the rapid evolution of simulation-based education makes it critical that approved programs have mechanisms to continually enhance their educational effectiveness based on feedback loops from participants and on ongoing research. For approval, the program application must also include a description of the educational offerings and how they are developed, proof of instructor competency and program leadership, the availability of CME credit, and adequate educational technology and infrastructure to support the courses offered. Programs must also indicate how they plan to ensure confidentiality of participants, and how they will manage conflict among participants and complaints about courses or instructors. Site visits by reviewers will initially occur on a random, rotating basis. Each program or center will pay application fees to the ASA to support site visits, making this ASA-sponsored system revenue neutral.

ASA Committee on Simulation Education headed by Randy Steadman

At the 2006 meeting of the ASA in Chicago, the ASA House of Delegates formally sanctioned the formation of the new ASA Committee on Simulation Education, based on the recommendation of the ASA Workgroup on Simulation Education. Randy Steadman was appointed chair of this new committee. Members were appointed from a list of qualified volunteers to serve as part of the committee assigned to initiate ASA-endorsed courses throughout the United States (see Table 1). To ensure that endorsed programs have appropriate faculty, facilities, and content to serve the needs of ASA members, a subcommittee plans to begin application review in 2007. Requirements for Maintenance of Certification in Anesthesiology will include simulation-based education or assessment for all graduates of the year 2007 and beyond. Thus, the ASA is encouraging the development of simulation-based programs and enticing members to take advantage of them. Standard courses may be developed within subspecialty societies for distribution to approved simulation centers.

Related and concurrent events

Several other groups and organizations are also engaged in developing simulation-based education and assessment. Spawned from simulation interest groups within anesthesiology, the Society for Simulation in Healthcare has evolved into a multidisciplinary, multispecialty, international organization dedicated to the advancement of all types of simulation-based education and advances in health care [32]. Another group, Advanced Initiatives in Medical Simulation, has taken on the task of lobbying the United States government for additional funding for health care simulation research and development [33]. Accrediting bodies are exploring simulation in earnest to determine its role in evaluation and testing. Some forms of simulation, such as simulation using standardized patients, are already well entrenched in the testing and credentialing systems, such as the US Medical Licensing Examination [34]. The American Board of Internal Medicine will possibly begin requiring assessment of cardiac catheterization skills using simulators for subspecialty certification in interventional cardiology [35]. A plan by the American College of Surgeons has also developed standards that delineate what the college calls Comprehensive Education Institutes, which focus on simulation-based education for members, providing additional incentives for the development and dissemination of simulation-based CME and, ultimately, surgical residency training [36]. Other organizations are developing standards for their own constituents. Most current users of simulation-based health care education are in the nursing and paramedical fields, with a large number in the military.

Despite the early work by anesthesiologists using simulation-based teaching and practice, simulation-based CME is rarely available for advanced anesthesiology training. This is likely due to a number of factors, including the additional cost, the increased effort (both of participants and faculty), and the inadequate equipment and course offerings for simulation-based CME compared with those for conventional CME. Another factor that may be critical is the fear of practicing professionals that they will be embarrassed or humiliated as they care for a simulated patient. Despite the potential barriers, many believe that simulation for some types of learning provides education that is superior to that obtained from a traditional lecture or journal format. Simulation-based teaching more closely mimics clinical teaching where the thought process is similar to that used when in clinical medicine. The stress of a simulated environment may improve the learning that occurs by evoking emotion that improves recall. It is also possible that simulated environments push students to a point where they are paralyzed with fear (Fig. 3) [37]. Simulation instructors typically take great pains to reassure students that the simulated environment is a "safe" place to learn, which means it is also a place where mistakes can be made without serious consequences. The best simulation-based teaching requires a careful balance between the stress of a real clinical experience and the safety of a classroom. As many educators have acknowledged, there is no learning without emotion.

Summary

With simulation-based education expanding at a rapid, almost frenetic pace, it is difficult to predict the future of such education. Ultimately, the underlying purpose is to approach learning and testing in an environment that is similar to actual practice. It is hoped that this approach will more accurately guide and predict behavior in actual practice, but this has not actually been proven. Demonstrating that one *can* perform well in a simulated environment does not guarantee that one *will* perform well in an actual case. On the other hand, many have already accepted the converse: If one is unable to perform well in a simulated environment, one will be unlikely to perform well in real cases either. This again is not yet proven, but

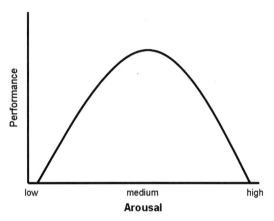

Fig. 3. Graph of Yerkes-Dodson Law principle. (*From* Wikipedia. Available at: http://en.
wikipedia.org/wiki/Yerkes-Dodson_law. Accessed October 26, 2004.)

evidence is accumulating that simulation may be at least as reasonable as
previous teaching methods and assessment tools, such as residency training
and board examinations. Given the strong impetus by multiple diverse organizations, many predict that simulation-based teaching will generate the
next revolution in health care education. The ASA is hoping to capitalize
on anesthesiology's long involvement and leadership in simulation-based
health care education to help bring about this revolution.

Appendix 1

Simulation program terms

Application. Written materials submitted by a program as part of its re-
quest for ASA approval.

Approval. The designation of a simulation program as one that provides
high-quality simulation courses to ASA members and that results from
a formal evaluation process conducted by the ASA through a committee on simulation education. Approvals will be time-limited.

Center. A well-organized entity where simulation courses are taught. A
center typically is based in a dedicated physical facility that has the infrastructure necessary to conduct simulation activities. A center may
support several simulation programs.

Committee. The ASA Committee on Simulation Education whose responsibilities, outlined in this document, include approval of simulation programs.

Course. A circumscribed educational experience, based on well-defined
educational objectives, that uses simulation as a primary tool for meeting these objectives. In this document, a course is specifically one
intended for ASA members.

Course director. An ASA member with documented knowledge, expertise, qualifications, responsibility, and authority to lead a specific course.

Criteria. Specific attributes of a simulation program that determine its ability to provide high-quality courses. The ability of a program to demonstrate that it meets criteria established by the Committee is the basis for approval.

Educational technology. All types of simulators, audiovisual equipment, clinical equipment and supplies, computers, software (eg, for scheduling, assessment, debriefing, video archiving), and other equipment and props that support a program's educational activities.

Instructor. An individual with documented knowledge and expertise in simulation education who teaches courses within a program.

Program. An identifiable entity whose primary mission is to provide simulation courses and other simulation-based activities. A program is defined by the courses it offers. Thus, programs are typically specific to a discipline or training process. A program can exist within a center or be independent. An anesthesiology program may contain courses, for example, on pain management, anesthesia crisis resource management, critical care support, difficult airway management, resuscitation, or cardiac ultrasonography.

Program director. An individual with documented knowledge, expertise, qualifications, responsibility, and authority to lead a simulation program.

Appendix 2

Nine basic criteria for program approval

Mission statement. The application should describe the program's mission in general and specifically with regard to simulation courses.

Educational offerings. The program should describe in detail the courses it intends to offer. The description of each course should include information about educational objectives, curriculum, evaluation methods, instructors, logistics, annual capacity, and projected cost. Information specifically about capacity could include, for example, the intended number of courses to be offered annually and the number of ASA members who could be accommodated per course. In addition, the application should describe the history of all of the program's courses over the last 2 years, including course evaluations.

Curriculum and scenario development process. The program should have an established curriculum development process that includes objectives, methods, and evaluations. Similarly, the program should have a scenario development process based on a standard template. The application should include a sample course curriculum and scenario.

Instructor competency. The program should have a process for training, evaluating, and credentialing its instructors. This process should address the attributes of simulation teaching expertise, scholarship in simulation and medical education principles, and expertise in the assigned course subject matter. The application should provide clear documentation that (1) at least one instructor in each course meets the program's credentialing standards and (2) at least one instructor in each course is an ABA-certified anesthesiologist.

Program leadership. The program should be administered by a designated program director who is responsible for the organization, conduct, and quality of the program. The program director should hold a doctoral degree and have an academic appointment at an accredited educational institution. Courses should be administered by a designated course director responsible for the conduct and quality of the course. Where appropriate, the program director and course director may be the same person. The course director should be credentialed as an instructor by the program, hold a doctoral degree, have an appointment in a department of anesthesiology of an accredited educational institution, and be an ASA member.

CME credits. The program should provide CME credit for its courses. CME credit may be granted by the program itself, by an affiliated educational institution, or through accredited outside entities, such as the ASA. Note that approval does not obligate the ASA to provide CME credit for a program's course; that is a separate approval process.

Assessing course effectiveness. The program should have a reliable process for the evaluation by trainees of courses and instructors. The evaluation process should document the effectiveness of each course in achieving its stated educational objectives. The program should have an internal quality-assurance process for both courses and instructors. The application will document the process for implementing changes in response to unsatisfactory evaluation data.

Educational technology. The program should have the educational technology necessary to effectively conduct its intended courses. The application should describe the available educational technology, how it is used, and how it is maintained and supported.

Infrastructure. The program should have an infrastructure sufficient to assure consistent high-quality courses. The infrastructure includes governance, fiscal viability, facilities, personnel, organizational relationships, policies and procedures, and capacity.

    a. *Governance and fiscal issues.* The program should be organized to maximize the likelihood that course quality will be maintained for the duration of the approval. The program should have standard and auditable processes for managing course income. The application should provide documentation of the program's governance and financial model, including evidence of stable program leadership and finances. Principal stakeholders in the program and its affiliated center or centers should be listed as well as their proportional usage of the facilities

b. *Facilities and capacity*. The program should have sufficient facilities and instructional capacity to consistently offer its courses. The application should describe the program's facilities, including physical layout and dimensions, available personnel, technical capabilities, and the typical flow of course participants within the facility during a course. Capacity refers to the affiliated facility's size and current percentage use for courses as well as all other activities. Other issues, such as registration and scheduling processes, and course participant management (eg, parking, meals) should be addressed in the application.

c. *Policies and procedures*. The program should have established written policies and procedures. Policies and procedures should address how courses are to be conducted, mechanisms to ensure quality instruction, maintenance of trainee confidentiality, trainee refunds and cancellations, and remedies in the event of conflicts. Compliance with applicable governmental and other regulations should be documented.

References

[1] History of the Safar Center for Resuscitation Research. Available at: http://www.safar. pitt.edu/content/archive/history/index_history.html. Accessed May 15, 2007.
[2] Tjomsland N. From stavanger with care: Laerdals first 50 years. Stavanger (Norway): Laerdal; 1990.
[3] Tjomsland N. Saving more lives—together. Stavanger (Norway): Laerdal; 2005.
[4] Abrahamson S. Human simulation for training in anesthesiology. Year Book Medical Publishers, Inc.; 1974. p. 370–4.
[5] Abrahamson S. Sim One—a patient simulator ahead of its time. Caduceus 1997;13:29–41.
[6] Abrahamson S. An interview of Professor Stephen Abrahamson. Educ Health (Abingdon) 2003;16:378–84.
[7] Abrahamson S, Denson JS, Wolf RM. Effectiveness of a simulator in training anesthesiology residents. 1969. Qual Saf Health Care 2004;13:395–7.
[8] Denson JS, Abrahamson S. A computer-controlled patient simulator. JAMA 1969;208: 504–8.
[9] Abrahamson S, Denson JS, Clark AP, et al. Anesthesiological training simulator. Edited by Office US Patent Office. USA; 1970.
[10] Doyle D, Arellano R. The virtual anesthesiology training simulation system [editorial]. Can J Anaesth 1995;42:267–73.
[11] Gaba DM, DeAnda A. A comprehensive anesthesia simulation environment: re-creating the operating room for research and training. Anesthesiology 1988;69:387–94.
[12] Holzman RS, Cooper JB, Gaba DM, et al. Anesthesia crisis resource management: real-life simulation training in operating room crises. J Clin Anesth 1995;7:675–87.

[13] Gaba DM. Human error in anesthetic mishaps. Int Anesthesiol Clin 1989;27(3):137–47.

[14] Howard SK, Gaba DM, Fish KJ, et al. Anesthesia Crisis Resource Management Training: teaching anesthesiologists to handle critical incidents. Aviat Space Environ Med 1992.

[15] Schwid HA, O'Donnell D. The Anesthesia Simulator-Recorder: a device to train and evaluate anesthesiologists' responses to critical incidents. Anesthesiology 1990;72:191–7.

[16] Schwid HA, O'Donnell D. Anesthesiologists' management of simulated critical incidents. Anesthesiology 1992;76:495–501.

[17] Hallinan JT. Heal thyself; once seen as risky, one group of doctors changes its ways;anesthesiologists now offer model of how to improve safety, lower premiums; surgeons are following suit. New York: Wall Street Journal; 2005. p. 1.

[18] Pierce EC. The 34th Rovenstein Lecture: forty years behind the mask: safety revisited, Available at: http://www.apsf.org/about/rovenstine. Accessed May 15, 2007.

[19] Siker ES. APSF History. Available at: http://www.apsf.org/about/brief_history.mspx. Accessed May 15, 2007.

[20] Seymour NE, Gallagher AG, Roman SA, et al. Virtual reality training improves operating room performance: results of a randomized, double-blinded study. Ann Surg 2002;236: 458–63 [discussion: 463–4].

[21] Blum MG, Powers TW, Sundaresan S. Bronchoscopy simulator effectively prepares junior residents to competently perform basic clinical bronchoscopy. Ann Thorac Surg 2004;78: 287–91 [discussion: 287–91].

[22] Colt HG, Crawford SW, Galbraith O 3rd. Virtual reality bronchoscopy simulation: a revolution in procedural training. Chest 2001;120:1333–9.

[23] Moorthy K, Smith S, Brown T, et al. Evaluation of virtual reality bronchoscopy as a learning and assessment tool. Respiration 2003;70:195–9.

[24] Andreatta PB, Woodrum DT, Birkmeyer JD, et al. Laparoscopic skills are improved with LapMentor training: results of a randomized, double-blinded study. Ann Surg 2006;243: 854–60 [discussion: 860–3].

[25] Haque S, Srinivasan S. A meta-analysis of the training effectiveness of virtual reality surgical simulators. IEEE Trans Inf Technol Biomed 2006;10:51–8.

[26] Goldmann K, Steinfeldt T. Acquisition of basic fiberoptic intubation skills with a virtual reality airway simulator. J Clin Anesth 2006;18:173–8.

[27] US Food and Drug Administration Center for Devices and Radiological Health, Medical Devices Advisory Committee, Circulatory System Devices Panel meeting. Edited by FDA. Gaithersburg (MD), April 21, 2004. Available at: http://www.fda.gov/ohrms/dockets/ac/04/transcripts/4033t1.htm. Accessed May 15, 2007.

[28] Gallagher AG, Cates CU. Approval of virtual reality training for carotid stenting: what this means for procedural-based medicine. JAMA 2004;292:3024–6.

[29] Cooke M, Irby DM, Sullivan W, et al. American medical education 100 years after the Flexner Report. N Engl J Med 2006;355:1339–44.

[30] Institute of Medicine. To err is human: building a safer health system. Washington, DC, Available at: http://www.nap.edu/books/0309068371/html. National Academy Press, 2000. Accessed May 15, 2007.

[31] ASA Member Poll on Simulation CME Statistics. Available at: http://www.asahq.org/SIM/memberpollstats040606.pdf. 2006. Accessed May 15, 2007.

[32] Society for Simulation in Healthcare. Available at: http://ssih.org. Accessed May 15, 2007.

[33] Advanced Iniatives in Medical Simulation. Available at: http://www.medsim.org/index.asp. Accessed May 15, 2007.

[34] United States Medical Licensing Examination. Available at: http://www.usmle.org/default.asp. Accessed May 15, 2007.

[35] American Board of Internal Medicine-Interventional Cardiology. Available at: http://www.abim.org/cert/policies_aqic.shtm. Accessed May 15, 2007.

[36] American College of Surgeons Division of Education Accredited Education Institutes. Available at: http://www.facs.org/education/accreditationprogram/index.html. Accessed May 15, 2007.
[37] Yerkes RM, Dodson JD. The relation of strength of stimulus to rapidity of habit-formation. Journal of Comparative Neurology and Psychology 1908;18:459–82.

ELSEVIER
SAUNDERS

ANESTHESIOLOGY
CLINICS

Anesthesiology Clin
25 (2007) 225–236

Does Simulation Improve Patient Safety?: Self-Efficacy, Competence, Operational Performance, and Patient Safety

Akira Nishisaki, MD[a,b,*], Ron Keren, MD, MPH[b,c],
Vinay Nadkarni, MD[a,d]

[a]Division of Critical Care, Department of Anesthesiology and Critical Care Medicine,
The Children's Hospital of Philadelphia, 34th Street and Civic Center Boulevard,
Philadelphia, PA 19104, USA
[b]Division of General Pediatrics, The Children's Hospital of Philadelphia, 3535 Market Street,
Room 1524, Philadelphia, PA 19104, USA
[c]Department of Pediatrics, University of Pennsylvania School of Medicine,
34th Street and Civic Center Boulevard, Philadelphia, PA 19104, USA
[d]Department of Anesthesiology and Critical Care, University of Pennsylvania School
of Medicine, 34th Street and Civic Center Boulevard, Philadelphia, PA 19104, USA

It has been more than 5 years since the Institute of Medicine (IOM) published "To Err Is Human," a report that raised public awareness about patient safety [1]. The IOM report estimated that each year 45,000 to 98,000 patients die in the United States as a result of medical error. The majority of these errors are the result of system problems rather than poor performance by particular individuals. The report called for systemic change in health care practices and highlighted the potential benefits of teamwork and simulation [1]. The Agency of Health Care Research and Quality (AHRQ) defines patient safety as "the absence of the potential for, or the occurrence of, health care associated injury to patients created by avoiding medical errors as well as taking action to prevent errors from causing injury" [2]. In response to the IOM report, the AHRQ implemented a broad

Akira Nishisaki and Vinay Nadkarni are supported by Agency for Healthcare Research and Quality grant 1U18HS 01667801. Vinay Nadkarni is an uncompensated scientific consultant for Laerdal Medical Co. and Medical Education and Technology Inc. (METI).

* Corresponding author. Division of Critical Care Medicine, The Department of Anesthesiology and Critical Care Medicine, The Children's Hospital of Philadelphia, 34th Street and Civic Center Boulevard, Philadelphia, PA 19104.

E-mail address: nishisaki@email.chop.edu (A. Nishisaki).

doi:10.1016/j.anclin.2007.03.009
anesthesiology.theclinics.com

and diverse patient safety initiative, including funding for simulation research with the understanding that simulation can complement other organizational change methods to facilitate adoption and implementation of best practices and technologies.

Simulation is defined as a strategy or technique to mirror or amplify real clinical situations with guided experiences in an interactive fashion [3,4]. By comparison, a simulator refers to a physical object or representation on which the full or partial task is replicated during the simulation [5]. High-fidelity simulation uses simulators that change and respond to the users and trainees. These include realistic three-dimensional procedural simulators, interactive simulators, and virtual reality simulators [6].

In this article, the authors review (1) the role of simulation to improve patient safety; (2) evidence for the effectiveness of simulation exercises to improve health care provider self-efficacy, competence, operational performance, and patient outcomes; and (3) future directions for simulation in healthcare.

Role of simulation in improvement of patient safety

Health care as a high-hazard industry

Health care, especially the complex hospital care required to treat serious diseases, falls into the category of a high-hazard industry like aviation, chemical manufacturing, nuclear power generation, and the military. Intensive research has gone into improving safety in these high-hazard industries. The two most dominant theories for understanding accidents in high-hazard industries are the Normal Accidents Theory and the High Reliability Organization Theory [7–9].

The Normal Accidents Theory focuses on the complexity of a system and the tight coupling of the interactions between components as a systematic root of accidents in high-hazard industries. When a problem cascade starts and all the holes in the barriers to accident prevention line up (described as the "Swiss cheese" model) (Fig. 1) [10], an accident occurs [7,11,12]. Health care systems are complex and hospitals exhibit tight coupling when processes are intrinsically time-sensitive once a process is set in motion [7]. For example, when a decision is made to do any therapeutic intervention, such as administration of a drug on a patient, tight time constraints mean that few checkpoints are in place to guard against a mistake [12].

Meanwhile, according to the High Reliability Organization Theory, the proper organization of people, technology, and processes can accommodate complex and hazardous activities at an acceptable level of performance [7–9]. This theory asserts that high numbers of operations, intensive training of personnel and teams, and intensive critiques of performance during operations and training support a culture of reliability and prepare the work group for future operations. However, even a high volume of routine

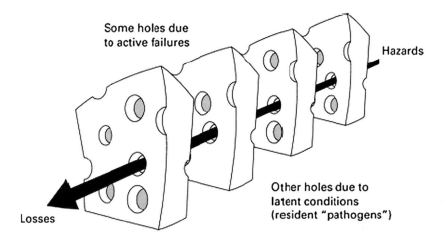

Successive layers of defences, barriers and safeguards

Fig. 1. The Swiss cheese metaphor for the genesis of medical mishaps in a complex environment. (*From* Reason JT, Carthey J, de Leval MR. Diagnosing "vulnerable system syndrome": an essential prerequisite to effective risk management. Qual Health Care 2001;10:ii21; with permission.)

operations may not prepare the organization for all circumstances it must handle. To counteract the complacency that comes from routine activities and to prepare for unexpected events, crews are trained intensively in drills and simulations for unusual situations [7].

Role of simulation training to improve patient safety

In the High Reliability Organization model, simulation training to improve patient safety may need to occur in a micro-system first [9,13]. As defined by the IOM, operating rooms, intensive care units, and individual nursing units are micro-systems that are small and functioning autonomously within a larger macro-system, which is typically a hospital. Simulation training can be used in micro-systems for a number of reasons including, but not limited to,

Routine training for emergencies
Training for teamwork
Establishing an environment for discussing errors without punishment
Testing new procedures for safety
Evaluating competence
Testing usability of devices
Investigating human performance
Providing skills training for novices outside of the production environment [9]

Training for teamwork is of particular importance for two reasons. First, medical care has become more complicated and requires a multidisciplinary approach. This is especially true in acute care areas, such as operating rooms and intensive care units [14]. This multidisciplinary approach is advocated to improve quality of care and patient safety by such professional organizations as the Society of Critical Care Medicine [15,16].

Second, although this multidisciplinary approach is routinely required in patient care, most medical education and training is still provided in "silos" inside of each discipline. While fundamental knowledge is required in each discipline, to function as a crew, team training with clear objectives to achieve best team performance cuts across all disciplines and is essential to improve patient safety [17]. This training is best provided by high-fidelity simulation in health care [17–19]. This is further discussed in the articles in this issue by Sundar and colleagues and by Hunt and colleagues.

Fidelity of simulation as an educational tool

High fidelity is achieved either by improving physical fidelity (ie, through a training device that replicates the physical characteristics of the real task) or by functional fidelity (ie, through a simulated task requiring skills that closely match those needed for the real task) [20]. The degree of fidelity desired for the training depends on the objectives of the training. A task trainer may be sufficient for teaching skills to individuals at the beginner's level. However, a high-fidelity simulation is typically more effective in crew resource management training (ie, team training), or for more advanced training, such as vascular stent placement [20,21]. For training in acute care areas, such as intensive care settings where initial management and therapeutic interventions are critical, high-fidelity simulation is becoming the training tool of choice because it can simulate real critical-care events. The use of high-fidelity simulation appears to be increasingly common, as evidenced by the rapid increase in simulation-related health care publications in the last few years [6] and the proliferation of simulation programs worldwide. Features of high-fidelity simulation training associated with effective learning are shown in Table 1 [6].

Does simulation improve patient safety?

To answer the question of whether simulation improves patient safety, we will use a conceptual framework based on Miller's [22] four levels of medical skill assessment [23] and Issenberg's system for classifying effectiveness of learning [6]. Our framework consists of four key elements: self-efficacy, competence, operational performance, and patient outcome.

Self-efficacy

Self-efficacy is a cognitive mechanism based on expectations or beliefs about one's ability to perform actions necessary to produce a given effect.

Table 1
Features of high-fidelity simulation training associated with effective learning

Features of simulation-based education	Percent of journal articles highlighted this feature
Providing feedback	47%
Repetitive practice	39%
Curriculum integration	25%
Range of difficulty level	14%
Multiple learning strategies	10%
Capture clinical variation	10%
Controlled environment	9%
Individualized learning	9%
Defined outcomes	6%
Simulator validity	3%

Data from Issenberg SB, McGaghie WC, Petrusa ER, et al. Features and uses of high-fidelity medical simulation that lead to effective learning: a BEME systematic review. Med Teach 2005;27:10–28.

In simulation-based assessment and training, self-efficacy is a trainee's degree of confidence in performing a procedure or in providing patient care evaluated by self-assessment in the face of simulation. Reznek and colleagues [24] demonstrated that a crisis resource management course with high-fidelity simulation improved self-efficacy for emergency medicine residents in crisis management. In a simulation-based orientation training for first-year pediatric critical-care fellows in the United States, students viewed simulation training for common pediatric critical-care management as effective for improving self-efficacy [25]. In a simulation-based training of study coordinators for a clinical research protocol, high-fidelity simulation training was effective in significantly improving confidence in affective, cognitive, and psychomotor domains [26].

Although self-efficacy is not difficult to assess and improve, no consistent correlation with observed measures of competence can be found [27]. Leopold and colleagues [28] measured a correlation between self-assessment and objective performance of arthrocentesis on a simple task trainer as a part of continuous medical education. They reported an inverse correlation between self-assessment and competence before the training ($r = -0.253$, $P = .02$). In the post-training evaluation, there was a positive correlation ($r = 0.24$, $P = .04$). Moorthy and colleagues [29] tested the correlation between self-assessment and objective ratings by experts (ie, competence) in technical and nontechnical skills in 27 surgical residents at three different training levels. Surgical trainees encountered a hypoxic event when a surgical procedure (saphenofenoral high-tie) was performed on a synthetic model attached to a high-fidelity simulator in an operating theater. The correlation of self-efficacy measurements with actual technical skills was weak (0.24) for junior trainees, but improved with increasing experience. There was a low correlation between the self-assessment and the expert scores in human factor skills, such as communication and leadership, during the crisis.

Overall, there is good evidence that simulation education can improve individual and team confidence and self-efficacy. It is not clear how simulation education compares with education through traditional didactic training groups in terms of self-efficacy improvement. The correlation between confidence or self-efficacy and observed measures of competence is not consistent [28] and may be affected by training level [30].

Competence

Competence is a capability to perform a particular professional task with an acceptable level of skill. In the context of medical simulation, competence is the degree to which simulation training objectively improves a trainee's ability to perform a procedure or provide patient care. Many simulation-related studies measure competence to some extent. In a high-fidelity simulation training in the acute care setting, this evaluation of competence is typically based on video-captured images and sounds with at least two independent raters. This measurement is done either by a detailed checklist or global scoring by trained experts in the field.

Multiple studies in procedural simulators, such as surgical, obstetric or laparoscopic simulators, suggest that simulation training can increase trainee competence [31–35]. A few studies suggest simulation training in acute care settings can improve individual or team competence. Rosenthal and colleagues [36] reported the effectiveness of high-fidelity simulation training on emergency airway management. After a pretest, 49 first-year medicine residents were trained with high-fidelity simulation either by a critical care attending or by a senior house staff member. Six weeks after the training, they were retested with simulation. Their emergency airway competence significantly improved in both groups regardless of the trainer's level.

A recent report documented that simulation-based training was superior to problem-based learning (PBL) for acquisition of critical assessment and management skills in medical students. In this study, 31 students were randomized to simulation training group or PBL group. Their assessment and management skills in critical respiratory scenarios were evaluated with checklists before and after the training. Evaluation was done with high-fidelity simulation. The simulation group performed significantly better than the PBL group [37].

The effect of simulation training on team competence for crisis management was evaluated in radiology residents. Twenty-four radiology residents were trained with high-fidelity simulation using two crisis scenarios. The scores in global assessment, use of support personnel, and use of resources significantly improved after the simulation training [38]. In an evaluation by DeVita and colleagues [19,39] of crisis management team training in acute care settings, the efficacy of high-fidelity simulation training on clinical competence was measured in terms of simulator survival rate and task completion rate. The team performance showed improvement in overall simulation survival rate and task completion rate from 0% to 90% and 31% to 89%, respectively.

Knowledge regarding the reliability and validity of simulation-based competence assessment is accumulating. Boulet and colleagues [40] assessed the clinical competence of 13 residents and 24 medical students with high-fidelity simulation in acute care settings. Each participant encountered six scenarios. The session was videotaped and clinical competence was rated by two to four expert raters. They found inter-rater reliability of simulation-based assessments was moderate and most influenced by the choice and number of simulation scenarios. The validity of simulation scores was supported by the positive correlation between trainees' performance and their clinical background and experience. Murray and colleagues [41] tested anesthesiology residents' acute care skills with high-fidelity simulation. They reported the inter-rater reliability was high among raters expert in the field and the overall global evaluation was more reproducible than the traditional checklist scoring method.

Overall, there is good evidence that simulation-based assessment can measure clinical competence with good reliability and validity. There is good evidence that simulation-based education can improve procedural and crew resource management competence in the simulation site.

Simulation and operational performance

Operational performance is a detailed examination of observable clinical assessment or therapeutic intervention associated with the execution or completion of a required clinical task in an actual clinical setting. Operational performance measures should ideally be able to quantify the degree to which competent care in simulation training sessions translates into competence in real clinical care settings. Operational performance can be assessed in terms of process of care measurements that are likely to be associated with clinical outcome.

Few studies have measured the efficacy of medical simulation training on operational performance in clinical settings. Mayo and colleagues [42] evaluated the effectiveness of high-fidelity simulation training on competence and operational performance of initial emergency airway management by first-year medical residents. Operational performance in emergency airway management in actual clinical settings was followed for 10 months after the training. Mayo and colleagues reported excellent performance by residents with high correct performance rate (91–100%), although there was no control group. At least four randomized controlled trials (RCTs) have demonstrated the effectiveness of high-fidelity procedural simulation to improve operational performance for endoscopic or surgical procedures. In an RCT involving virtual reality colonoscopy, 10 surgeons and 2 medical gastroenterologists who had experience with endoscopy but not colonoscopy were trained either by high-fidelity simulation plus standard training (a booklet and an instructive CD) or by standard training only. The simulation training group had a significantly higher rate of intubation of the cecum (52%) in comparison to the standard training group (19%) in initial 10 colonoscopies on actual patients [43]. In an RCT of a virtual reality laparoscopy simulation training, 16 surgical residents (post-graduate year one through four) were trained either by high-fidelity simulation plus standard surgical residency training or by a standard training only. All residents performed laparoscopic cholecystectomy with an attending surgeon blinded to each resident's training status. Gallbladder resection was 29% faster and five times less likely to burn nontarget tissue in the high-fidelity simulation training group [44]. Grantcharov and colleagues [45] reported a similar RCT of virtual reality laparoscopy simulation training for 20 surgical residents. Surgeons who received simulation training performed laparoscopic cholecystectomy significantly faster than the control group. Finally, in an RCT of high-fidelity catheter-based simulation training, 20 surgical residents without previous endovascular experience received either standard didactic training for the technique of catheter intervention for angioplasty or standard training with an additional 2 hours of high-fidelity simulation training. Within 2 weeks, resident performance was evaluated on femoral or iliac angioplasty in actual clinical settings. The simulation group was significantly more successful in completing cases and showed higher scores on a procedural checklist and on a global rating scale [46].

No clinical trials of simulation training for a medical team have been performed to demonstrate improved operational performance in clinical settings.

Overall, there is good evidence that procedural simulation improves operational performance in actual clinical settings. However, no evidence yet shows that simulation training for crew resource management actually improves operational performance at the bedside. Much more data about the implementation and transferability of classroom simulations on actual patient care are required.

Simulation and patient outcome

To date, no direct evidence has demonstrated that simulation training improves actual patient safety outcomes. Research is sorely needed in this area. Studying the effect of simulation on patient outcomes has been difficult in the past because, with a small number of poor outcomes at baseline, a large number of subjects (trainees) is necessary to show a difference in patient outcome. Furthermore, it is difficult to avoid contamination in conducting a trial of a large educational intervention.

Future directions

Although the number of simulation centers built in the United States and other countries is increasing, many physicians remain unfamiliar with them because they have not had time to use them or because the nearest center is too far away [45]. Nonetheless medical simulation training for individuals and medical teams to improve patient safety will continue to increase. As it does, its effect on operational performance and patient outcome needs to be vigorously evaluated. Simulation training will be used more in multidisciplinary team training as team performance is increasingly recognized as important in health care. New health care domains for applying simulation continue to be found. Such domains include the areas of clinical research coordinator education [26], research protocol feasibility evaluation [47], and in-service training in the use of new anesthetic devices [48].

Although low patient numbers may never permit the ultimate measure of training effectiveness—the impact of each simulation training on individual patient outcome—an evaluation may be possible of the effect of simulation on patient outcomes throughout an entire health care micro-system or macro-system. To achieve this, frequent crisis team competence assessment and crew resource management training by a simulation should be incorporated into patient safety initiatives.

New simulation technologies, such as virtual patients and advanced procedural trainers, are emerging. These are described in detail in the articles in this issue by Banerjee and colleagues, Patel and colleagues, Rudolph and colleagues, and Cantrell and colleagues. New training strategies, such as "just-in-time" training or "just-in-place" training, will be tested with this high-fidelity simulation technology. A mobile high-fidelity simulation cart or an on-site simulation room will facilitate this process [49].

Summary

Simulation training is an essential educational strategy for health care systems to improve patient safety. The strength of simulation training, especially high-fidelity simulation, is its suitability for multidisciplinary team training. There is good evidence that simulation training improves provider and team self-efficacy and competence on manikins. There is also good evidence that procedural simulation improves operational performance. However, no evidence yet shows that simulation training for crew resource management improves team operational performance in clinical settings. Furthermore, no evidence to date proves that simulation training actually improves patient outcome. Even so, confidence is growing in the validity of medical simulation as the training tool of the future. The use of medical simulation will continue to grow in the context of multidisciplinary team training for patient safety. The efficacy of simulation training on operational performance in clinical settings and patient outcome needs to be vigorously evaluated.

References

[1] Kohn L, Corrigan J, Donaldson M, editors. To error is human: building a safer health system. Washington, DC: National Academy Press; 1999.
[2] Pronovost PJ, Thompson DA, Holzmueller CG, et al. Defining and measuring patient safety. Crit Care Clin 2005;21:1–19.
[3] Improving Patient Safety through Simulation Research. Agency for healthcare research and quality. Available at: http://grants.nih.gov/grants/guide/rfa-files/RFA-HS-06-030.html. Accessed September 25, 2006.
[4] Gaba DM. The future vision of simulation in health care. Qual Saf Health Care 2004;13:2–10.
[5] Cooper JB, Taqueti VR. A brief history of the development of mannequin simulators for clinical education and training. Qual Saf Health Care 2004;13(Suppl 1):i11–8.
[6] Issenberg SB, McGaghie WC, Petrusa ER, et al. Features and uses of high-fidelity medical simulations that lead to effective learning: a BEME systematic review. Med Teach 2005;27:10–28.
[7] Gaba DM. Structural and organizational issues in patient safety. Calif Manage Rev 2000;43:83–102.
[8] AHRQ Patient Safety Network. A National Patient Safety Resource. Glossary. Available at: http://psnet.ahrq.gov/glossary.aspx. Accessed September 28, 2006.
[9] Cooper JB. The role of simulation in patient safety. In: Dunn WF, editor. Simulators in critical care and beyond. Des Plaines (IL): Society of Critical Care Medicine; 2004. p. 20–4.
[10] Perneger TV. The Swiss cheese model of safety incidents: are there holes in the metaphor? BMC Health Serv Res 2005;5:71.
[11] Dean B, Schachter M, Vincent C, et al. Causes of prescribing errors in hospital inpatients: a prospective study. Lancet 2002;359:1373–8.
[12] Duwe B, Fuchs BD, Hansen-Flaschen J. Failure mode and effects analysis application to critical care medicine. Crit Care Clin 2005;21:21–30.
[13] Slonim AD, Pollack MM. Integrating the Institute of Medicine's six quality aims into pediatric critical care: relevance and applications. Pediatr Crit Care Med 2005;6:264–9.
[14] Bion JF, Heffner JE. Challenges in the care of the acutely ill. Lancet 2004;363:970–7.
[15] Society of Critical Care Medicine Critical Care eNewsletter. Team building. Available at: http://sccmwww.sccm.org/publications/eNewsletters_Archive/01_20_2004.asp. Accessed September 27, 2006.
[16] Brilli RJ, Spevetz A, Branson RD, et al. Critical care delivery in the intensive care unit: defining clinical roles and the best practice model. Crit Care Med 2001;29:2007–19.
[17] Burke CS, Salas E, Wilson-Donnelly K, et al. How to turn a team of experts into an expert medical team: guidance from the aviation and military communities. Qual Saf Health Care 2004;13:96–104.
[18] Hamman WR. The complexity of team training: what we have learned from aviation and its applications to medicine. Qual Saf Health Care 2004;13(Suppl 1):i72–9.
[19] DeVita MA, Schaefer J, Lutz J, et al. Improving medical crisis team performance. Crit Care Med 2004;32(Suppl):S61–5.
[20] Maran NJ, Glavin RJ. Low- to high-fidelity simulation—a continuum of medical education? Med Educ 2003;37(Suppl 1):22–8.
[21] Dawson S. Procedural simulation: a primer. J Vasc Interv Radiol 2006;17:205–13.
[22] Miller GE. The assessment of clinical skills/competence/performance. Acad Med 1990;65(Suppl):s63–7.
[23] Epstein RM, Hundert EM. Defining and assessing professional competence. JAMA 2002;287:226–35.
[24] Reznek M, Smith-Coggins R, Howard S, et al. Emergency medicine crisis resource management (EMCRM): pilot study of a simulation-based crisis management course for emergency medicine. Acad Emerg Med 2003;10:386–9.

[25] Nishisaki A, Jarrah R, Biagas K, et al. A multi-institutional high fidelity simulation "Boot Camp" orientation and training program for pediatric critical care (PCC) fellows. Crit Care Med 2006;34:A121.

[26] Taekman JM, Hobbs G, Barber L, et al. Preliminary report on the use of high-fidelity simulation in the training of study coordinators conducting a clinical research protocol. Anesth Analg 2004;99:521–7.

[27] Davis DA, Mazmanian PE, Fordis M, et al. Accuracy of physician self-assessment compared with observed measures of competence. JAMA 2006;296:1094–102.

[28] Leopold SS, Morgan HD, Kadel NJ, et al. Impact of educational intervention on confidence and competence in the performance of a simple surgical task. J Bone Joint Surg Am 2005;87: 1031–7.

[29] Moorthy K, Munz Y, Adams S, et al. Self-assessment of performance among surgical trainees during simulated procedures in a simulated operating theater. Am J Surg 2006; 192:114–8.

[30] Gordon MJ. A review of the validity and accuracy of self-assessments in health professions training. Acad Med 1991;66:762–9.

[31] Ost D, DeRosiers A, Britt EJ, et al. Assessment of a bronchoscopy simulator. Am J Respir Crit Care Med 2001;164:2248–55.

[32] Fried MP, Satava R, Weghorst S, et al. Identifying and reducing errors with surgical simulation. Qual Saf Health Care 2004;13:19–26.

[33] Andreatta PB, Woodrum DT, Birkmeyer JD, et al. Laparoscopic skills are improved with LapMentor training. Ann Surg 2006;243:854–63.

[34] Aggarwal R, Black SA, Hance JR, et al. Virtual reality simulation training can improve inexperienced surgeons' endovascular skills. Eur J Vasc Endovasc Surg 2006;31:588–93.

[35] Deering S, Brown J, Hodor J, et al. Simulation training and resident performance of single-ton vaginal breech delivery. Obstet Gynecol 2006;107:86–9.

[36] Rosenthal ME, Adachi M, Ribaudo V, et al. Achieving housestaff competence in emergency airway management using scenario based simulation training. Chest 2006;129: 1453–8.

[37] Steadman RH, Coates WC, Huang YM, et al. Simulation-based training is superior to problem-based learning for acquisition of critical assessment and management skills. Crit Care Med 2006;34:151–7.

[38] Sica GT, Barron DM, Blum R, et al. Computerized realistic simulation: a teaching module for crisis management in radiology. AJR Am J Roentgenol 1999;172:301–4.

[39] DeVita MA, Schaefer J, Lutz J, et al. Improving medical emergency team (MET) performance using a novel curriculum and a computerized human patient simulator. Qual Saf Health Care 2005;14:326–31.

[40] Boulet JR, Murray D, Kras J, et al. Reliability and validity of a simulation-based acute care skills assessment for medical students and residents. Anesthesiology 2003;99: 1270–80.

[41] Murray DJ, Boulet JR, Kras JF, et al. Acute care skills in anesthesia practice. Anesthesiology 2004;101:1084–95.

[42] Mayo PH, Hackney JE, Mueck T, et al. Achieving house staff competence in emergency airway management: results of a teaching program using a computerized patient simulator. Crit Care Med 2004;32:2422–7.

[43] Ahlberg G, Hultcrantz R, Jaramillo E, et al. Virtual reality colonoscopy simulation: a compulsory practice for the future colonoscopist? Endoscopy 2005;37:1198–204.

[44] Seymour NE, Gallagher AG, Roman SA, et al. Virtual reality training improves operating room performance. Ann Surg 2002;236:458–64.

[45] Grantcharov TP, Kristiansen VB, Bendix J, et al. Randomized clinical trial of virtual reality simulation for laparoscopic skills training. Br J Surg 2004;91:146–50.

[46] Chaer RA, DeRubertis BG, Lin SC, et al. Simulation improves resident performance in catheter-based intervention. Ann Surg 2006;244:343–52.

[47] Wright MC, Taekman JM, Barber L, et al. The use of high fidelity human simulation as an evaluative tool in the development of clinical research protocols and procedures. Contemp Clin Trials 2005;26:646–59.
[48] Dalley P, Robinson B, Weller J, et al. The use of high-fidelity human patient simulation and the introduction of new anesthesia delivery systems. Anesth Analg 2004;99:1737–41.
[49] Weinstock PH, Kappus LJ, Kleinman ME, et al. Toward a new paradigm in hospital-based pediatric education: the development of an onsite simulator program. Pediatr Crit Care Med 2005;6:635–41.

ANESTHESIOLOGY
CLINICS

Anesthesiology Clin
25 (2007) 237–259

Simulation Applications for Human Factors and Systems Evaluation

Stephen D. Small, MD

Department of Anesthesiology and Critical Care, Center for Simulation and Safety in Healthcare, University of Chicago, 5806 South Blackstone Avenue, Chicago, IL 60637, USA

Simulation applications have become increasingly common in health care. A convergence of factors has stimulated this growth, including the rapid advance of enabling technologies, demand for improved outcomes and objectively assessed competencies, and translation of lessons learned from other high-risk industries as a function of the patient safety and quality movements. The bulk of the experience gained and resources expended has been focused on education, training, and assessment of clinicians' knowledge, skills, and attitudes. Point-of-care teams have been important targets of inquiry with interest in developing group-level performance measures, shaping teamwork curricula, and increasing transfer of training to actual care. Simulation methods also lend themselves to supporting human factors and systems-level investigations, yet work in health care has, to a large degree, been limited to a few experienced centers, interdisciplinary research teams, and isolated novel studies.

Excellent textbook references on human performance, safety, and human factors and simulation are available [1,2]. Much research in this emerging field has been introduced in preliminary abstracts and proceedings. A preliminary systematic search disclosed relevant papers of practical applications that have not been reviewed in this context. Several dimensions suggest potential useful commonalities. These include methods that might be generalized to other investigations in different clinical settings, approaches that could be added to other strategies to strengthen validity of research projects and provide additional insights, stimulation of additional research questions, and the strengthening of a social network of stakeholders with similar interests. In addition, the growing number of

This work was partially supported by Agency for Healthcare Research and Quality grant U18 HS016664-01.

E-mail address: ssmall@dacc.uchicago.edu

increasingly sophisticated medical simulation centers may find it in their interest to develop the capacity to engage in these types of studies for educational, safety, and quality improvement, or financial reasons.

This article structures the emerging literature base, discusses representative papers, and outlines opportunities and challenges. The chosen unit of analysis or focus is on interactions among clinicians, tools, tasks, patients, and the environment of clinical operations. Many definitions of "human factors" exist. The International Ergonomics Association provides the following definition:

> Ergonomics (or human factors) is the scientific discipline concerned with the understanding of interactions among humans and other elements of a system, and the profession that applies theory, principles, data and methods to design in order to optimize human well-being and overall system performance. Ergonomists contribute to the design and evaluation of tasks, jobs, products, environments and systems in order to make them compatible with the needs, abilities and limitations of people [3].

It is also useful to explicitly describe what is meant by "system." According to a common definition, a system is "a group of independent but interrelated elements comprising a unified whole" [4]. For our context, more specification is warranted. The concept of microsystems helps deliver that specification. The essential elements of a clinical microsystem are (1) a core team of healthcare professionals; (2) the defined population they care for; (3) an information environment to support the work of caregivers and patients; and (4) support staff, equipment, and a work environment [5]. It is also of interest to study larger components of the health care system, such as hospitals, networks, communities, or disease populations. Except for the case of realistic medical disaster management simulations using many volunteers, standardized patients, or manikins, "macro" level simulations may typically be performed as a computer-screen–based, fully digital exercise or study. While the field of large-scale digital computation is accelerating in health services research as well as in the biophysical sciences, this article is restricted to discussion of physical representation simulations, and suggests how those methods might relate to computational approaches.

No accepted definition of a health care "systems simulation" exists. Therefore, the following characteristics are proposed and may be refined. For practical purposes, health care simulations involving actual people, devices, and other artifacts of the work environment may be said to have a systems focus if (1) the simulation requires multiple patient representations, (2) the simulation enacts a clinical operational infrastructure for a task or tasks involving multiple clinicians or technicians with or without full patient representations, (3) a simulation of one or more patients extends over time to include movement across transitions in care settings or a series of tasks comprising an episode of care for a defined problem. These physical representations can be mapped to the three dimensions of complexity, scale, and organizational features.

The rationale behind defining a category of health care simulation dealing with systems is to acknowledge the unique elements and relationships that must be represented, the kinds of questions that might be asked, and the skills that require training. The essential characteristic is a scaling up from a single patient, clinician, device, task, or social analysis of a single team's issues to the next level of complexity in the organization and delivery of care. Fig. 1, based on concepts from ecological psychology, shows the different types and linkages of human factors and systems simulations.

Human performance

Full-scale simulation approaches have enabled investigators to study and probe aspects of human behavior that previously presented many ethical, logistical, and methodological barriers. Of course, simulator environments never completely present a 1:1 match to clinical reality in all cognitive, emotional, and psychomotor attributes. Also, with simulation, one cannot quantitatively assess the degree to which variation in

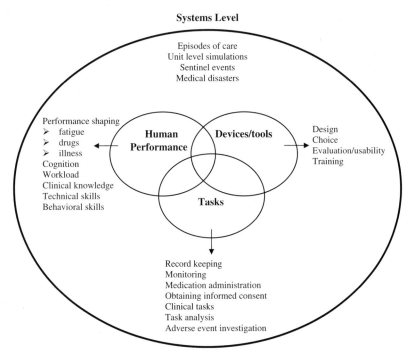

Fig. 1. Organization of simulation applications in human factors and systems investigation and training.

performance is a function of attributes of the individual, the presentation of the scenario as perceived by the individual (ie, invalid cues, sequencing), or an artifact of the participant's response to performing in a simulation and not an actual case with attendant risks. However, on the positive side, simulated scenarios with characteristics of interest can be standardized to a significant degree (eg, type of event, workload level, specific cues and challenges), presented on demand, and repeated. Also, with simulated scenarios, many kinds of data, including audiovisual data, can be easily captured.

The idea of a "stress test" has achieved commonplace status for decades in clinical medicine. Such tests involve giving adrenocorticotropin-releasing hormone to study cortisol response, or conducting a cardiac evaluation with physical or pharmacological stressors given intravenously to look at patterns of pump muscle and electrical function. Such stress tests allow us to systematically probe endocrine and organ system function to learn more about the capabilities and limits of their performance in a selective, graded, and fairly controlled manner. Both human performance and the domain of interest are so complex that it is usually necessary to constrain, limit, or alter the simulations in some manner to induce the behavior being studied, and to refrain from representing cues or tasks which reduce "useful signal/noise" ratios. Nonetheless the stress-test metaphor applies as simulation provides a medium to evaluate and augment the capability of systemic reserve to respond to stressors.

Participant self-reports of simulation realism and validity reported in the literature reflect the success of most immersion or high-fidelity staging. Although a relatively weak measure, this data confirms the anecdotal experience of experienced simulation instructors and researchers used to observing patterns of complex behavior during training simulations that mirror expectations from prior runs performed by others or comparisons to a trainee's clinical performances, or that produce patterns of responses similar to those seen in actual events from which simulation scenarios are sometimes scripted. More research on the ecological validity of full-scale simulations is needed.

Workload

Workload is composed of all tasks along all dimensions. For example, workload includes retrieval of information involving both long- and short-term memory. Workload also includes management of stress, which involves such issues as time pressure and interpersonal conflict. Workload also includes the task of juggling simultaneous and conflicting demands of changing priorities, such as dealing with cardiovascular variables while managing an unexpected difficult airway and intravenous access issues and requests for information. Experts are able to manage higher and more complex degrees of workload than those less experienced or able. In addition to having a larger, more varied base of experience to draw from, experts use such techniques as delegating tasks, delaying procedures, employing novel approaches, and taking shortcuts to succeed. Because challenge events can be standardized in simulations, studies in anesthesia simulations have replicated this finding. If experts do not perform as well as novices or the less experienced, questions will be raised as to the validity of the simulations. Medical experts are no different than chess experts, who do not have a recall edge over novices for piece positions if games are arranged randomly. As discussed below, poorly designed devices, workstations, or systems can increase workload.

Three overarching concepts are useful to review. First, there are essentially two ways to improve human performance: by training to improve skills and by redesigning tasks to make them easier. Second, reduction of workload frees up mental, physical, and emotional capacity to handle other tasks and allow more time for review, reflection, observation, and information-gathering. Third, studies of workload and task analysis can identify deficiencies in performance where training and, more importantly, task redesign can provide highly leveraged improvements in outcome. Mistakes tend to occur when some element of a system or task is hidden or unknown, leading to decisions based on guesses or to surprises that add complications. Mistakes also tend to occur during periods of sudden, high workload when (1) haste results in failure to complete tasks, failure to perform tasks in the proper sequence, or failure to properly record or transfer information, and (2) when a flood of data, such as noise from artifactual alarms, overwhelms normal decision-making processes and buries the most critical pieces of information. Full-scale training simulation scenarios are best designed with these elements in mind to induce behaviors of interest for debriefing and insure a naturalistic range of responses from trainees with different experience, decision-making styles and knowledge bases [6]. Simulation studies can also theoretically define and reproduce periods of high workload and help dissect the causes of performance deficiencies. Furthermore, such studies can be used to test novel techniques, refine them, and study them for possible unintended consequences, and eventually to conduct training on the use of the techniques (Fig. 2).

Detailed task analysis is usually performed in actual settings. The primary objective is not the induction of particular behaviors. In one classic study, researchers looked at such parameters as time taken for a task, number of tasks initiated, and subjective evaluations of workloads. They also measured spare mental capacity by proxy by capturing how often subjects noticed an artifactual probe light. The clinical setting was ambulatory surgical cases, and 11 third-year residents and 11 novice residents were studied. This work has been refined and expanded to include 32 task-categories [7]. Much of the research in this area has been presented in abstracts and does not involve simulation, although it has led to evaluation of graphical displays in full-scale simulators.

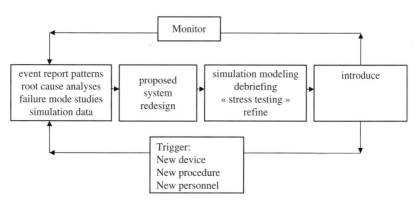

Fig. 2. Idealized model of simulation applications for systems design and improvement.

An exception is the more recent work of a European research group that aims to conduct these kinds of task analyses and workload and performance studies in an ecologically valid 1:1 simulated operating room and compare results with observations in actual clinical settings. The group developed a task analysis tool that has 41 codes, each representing an action, with an emphasis on capturing relationships between actions in time and function [8]. Major task groups included monitoring, measuring (typical anesthetic tasks), communicating, documenting, and performing additional operations (other anesthetic tasks and workplace and work crew interactions). In a preliminary report by the same group, six anesthesiologists were observed in two actual and three simulated cases. The task tool measured seven major groups of tasks, while also taking into account other activities under the "miscellaneous" category and recording when the anesthesiologist stepped out of the operating room. Two of the simulator cases involved scripted events [9]. With some exceptions, type of task and task-density were similar across measures, thus lending additional support for simulation validity, at least in that particular setting. The investigators pointed out that fewer tasks were required in the simulation environment, and emphasized organizational factors as important considerations for achieving ecological validity in simulation.

A recent extensive review of task, workload, vigilance, decision-making, and associated performance assessment techniques is available. Much promise exists for continuing to extend this work into full-scale simulation using more nuanced and complex scenarios, more ecologically valid simulation environments, and a wider range and larger number of practitioners.

Cognition in action

Another way to consider the potential of full-scale simulations is to focus on why clinicians fail, how they succeed, and how might expertise be augmented and shared without creating hazards to patients. This approach, perhaps a human factors approach, is an alternative to the use of full-scale simulations for assessing skills in managing the spectrum of typical anesthetic issues. Descriptive work studying the outcomes of clinicians' responses to simulated critical incidents has provided insights into the variability of performance even among experienced clinicians, and raised questions about how competency should be defined. Without data about clinicians' prior experiences, detailed debriefings, or systematic think-aloud protocols, however, understanding the why and how of performance, including simulation artifacts, is impossible. It matters whether the unit of analysis is the clinician or the man–machine–task system.

The concept of situation awareness is important in this regard. Situation awareness has been defined as "the perception of the elements in the environment within a volume of time and space, the comprehension of their meaning and the projection of their status in the near future" [10]. Situation awareness describes the formation and maintenance of the mental models practitioners use as bases for their decisions and actions [11]. Recent work is attempting to translate the apparent success of methods for measuring situation awareness in aviation and other domains to anesthesiology [12]. Simulation is a necessary component of some techniques to measure situation awareness. One such technique is the "freeze action—answer probe" method described in this paper. First, a task analysis and hierarchy of goals and actions is developed, followed by the creation of questions directed at increasing levels of situation awareness—perception, comprehension, and, the highest level, prediction of future states. The simulation is randomly interrupted, with guidelines for query length, time allowed for response, and total queries per simulation.

Only one recent paper has described the actual application of the situation awareness freeze-action technique in health care simulation [13]. This two-part study investigating the impact on situation awareness of two different monitor displays was problematic for several reasons. First, the simulation setting lacked significant ecological validity. Second, the number of queries was small, suggesting that participants might be able to predict the next question or type. Third, because investigators wanted subjects unfamiliar with the traditional monitor displays, the second part of the study used undergraduate college students who, compared to trained clinicians, probably lacked the professional motivation or risk boundaries for certain of the variables presented and their ranges. Finally, differences in time to perception of changes were not clinically significant and, in one case (bronchospasm), the time difference was so large as to suspect an artifact of the simulation itself, such as lack of presentation of usual cues or miscues.

The author has had personal experience piloting the situation awareness freeze-action method in an immersive simulation environment with skilled practitioners. The author found that the anesthesiologist subjects almost instantly adapted to simulation "freezes," typically studying the monitors before data streams ended. Multiple interruptions appeared intrusive.

Certain questions about the patient state (eg, location of prior coronary stents or type of cardiac surgery) could not be answered suddenly out of context after a brief turnover report, but were available when presented in the context of a relevant problem in the flow of the action. "Freezing" role-playing medical personnel in the environment introduced additional nuances not seen in cockpit-display situation-awareness studies.

Still, part of the lure of situation awareness measurement is the potential for using simulation to study alternative devices, designs, procedures, and training on clinicians' dynamic mental models. With more experience on how to design and carry out "live" situation awareness measures, the technique may prove useful, especially in combination with after-action debriefings, use of embedded probes in scenarios to elicit information more naturalistically, subjective workload measures, and other convergent techniques.

Performance-shaping factors

In studying human performance, researchers have long been interested in the effects of such factors as illness, fatigue, and medicines, including over-the-counter, illicit, and prescription drugs. Fatigue has received the most interest in full-scale simulation, although these studies are still scant because of the complexity and resource-intense nature of the exercises.

In the classic simulation study of rested versus sleep-deprived anesthesiologists, 12 residents performed anesthesia for laparoscopic surgery for 4 hours in a darkened room the morning after either restful sleep or no sleep [14]. Subjects were not allowed to consume caffeine in the 24-hour period before the simulations. Soft classical music played during the simulated surgeries and the operating room crews were instructed not to engage subjects in conversation. During the exercise, the subjects wore activity wristbands to validate sleep logs and other data. Meanwhile, simulation administrators monitored self-kept sleep logs, investigated the presence of any clinical sleep disorders, and surveyed preferences for morning or evening work. Halfway through the simulation, a 30-minute lunch break was provided in a place with normal lighting. In short, this was a study replete with elegant, well-thought-out controls, albeit presented in a rather extreme and somewhat artifactual situation, despite its seeming realism, presumably to leverage the impact of the sleep-deprived state.

Three types of task probes were presented to subjects to assess vigilance and spare mental capacity. One was a red on–off light not part of the clinical data stream. The other two were changes in two clinical monitor values. In addition, two clinical events were scripted to occur. Not surprisingly, sleep-deprived subjects caught up on their sleep during the delivery of anesthesia. However, task patterns and workload were not reported to be affected by lack of sleep, alertness conditions varied markedly over the duration of the case, and high intersubject variability obscured differences in time-to-corrective-action for events. Both groups picked up hidden faults in the anesthesia environment, and both made errors or took shortcuts in the preanesthetic machine check. The study was small due to its complexity and logistical barriers, such as having to perform the simulations on the daily circadian upswing in the late morning, and the rested group did not perform "near perfectly" as assumed.

What were the main take-home points of this important paper? First, large numbers of subjects are necessary to extend the findings of this research, which is challenging to do rigorously. Second, although the sleep-deprived subjects performed nearly as well as the rested subjects, sleep-deprived clinicians were not engaged in care during certain "outlier" events, such as when they were plainly sleeping for minutes at a time or taking "microsleeps." Theories of accident evolution and event cascade point to the presence of "triggering events," which are unusual and often singular convergences of irregularities that combine to push safety past thresholds where harm can occur. Although major failures did not occur in the simulations, the presence of sleeping and microsleeps coupled with decrements in mood, psychomotor vigilance, and memory in the sleep-deprived group created significant hazards.

Will there be additional in-depth, well-controlled, simulation-based studies of sleep and fatigue effects on human performance in health care? The absence of such studies speaks to their expense and complexity and to the potential limitations on findings. In the United States, work-hour regulations have been in effect for several years, but more action on this front can be anticipated given status of work hours for physicians in Europe and the lack of any restrictions on nonresident clinicians in the United States. Still, work-restricted clinicians have been shown not to use their extra time to sleep, but to moonlight or take on other duties, either personal or professional. Testing other measures to address the problem of fatigue, such as taking short naps, using caffeine or other accepted drugs, and restricting tired workers to less risky tasks, may create a need for evidence on which to base policy with far-reaching implications. Simulation research can help provide such evidence. The growth and increasing sophistication of simulation facilities may also enable rigorous simulation-based sleep and fatigue research to be performed by other disciplines responsible for taking care of patients in more distributed, extended settings, with greater need for communication and coordination and countermeasures for mood and memory deficits.

The study of prescription and over-the-counter drugs offers a new and important frontier for medical simulation. Many clinicians take beta-blockers, antidepressants, or other compounds that cross the blood–brain barrier and have known effects on performance. Beta-blockers classically affect the stress response and, theoretically, can improve or impair reaction times and other measures of performance by, for example, causing depression, which undermines performance, by decreasing impulsiveness, which may enhance performance, or by decreasing perceived stress, which can help or hurt performance. Many clinicians take antihistamines chronically or seasonally for allergies. Many also work while ill with flu syndromes or painful conditions compounded by fatigue and medications.

Strategic management simulations are lengthy, nuanced, table-top simulations in which participants receive an ongoing stream of computer-generated information about unfolding realistic events framed by a particular scenario for which they have received in-depth preparation for their roles [15]. Examples of scenarios include managing a company's affairs, dealing with a public health crisis, or coping with a disaster in a small town. The scenarios are characterized by complexity, change, ambiguity, and volatility, making them similar to the naturalistic decision-making school framework [16] used in full-scale medical simulation [6,17]. Strategic management simulations, which rely on low-technology tools but create highly realistic scenarios, are immersive to the extent that participants become deeply engaged. Data about decisions and actions are collected by computer to reduce bias, and integrated to provide 80 performance measures loading on 12 factors. Scores are produced reflecting complex information-processing attributes, such as activity, speed, responsiveness, initiative, breadth, planning, strategy, and emergency response. Validated results from large numbers of participants have shown the effects of sedatives, alcohol, caffeine, and cardiovascular medications on these higher level performance attributes [18–20]. Strategic management simulations have begun to be applied in health care training and assessment [21]. No studies were found using strategic management simulations or full-scale simulation to study the impact of factors shaping human performance in health care other than fatigue, discussed above.

Tasks

Monitoring

Monitoring is a key subtask in anesthesiology. This article discusses three papers about the use of simulation to evaluate clinicians' monitoring behaviors and the impact of newer displays over the past 10 years. An early classic study used simulation to investigate the impact of three currently used display formats on perception of changing physiological variables [22]. Measures of performance included response latency and accuracy. Participants included anesthesiology residents and college-educated lay people. The residents were allowed to become familiar with the displays by using a particular anesthesia machine and monitor, but all studies were conducted in a separate, nonclinical location using a computer-screen–based simulator. Anesthesia residents responded faster and with greater accuracy using the graphical displays than with numerical displays, but differences were so small as to preclude extrapolation to actual clinical work. Nonmedical participants performed less well than the residents, and did not appear to benefit from graphical displays. Although this study represents a highly artifactual, laboratory-controlled partial-task simulation, it helped introduce a new era of more sophisticated methods for studying human factors in anesthesiology.

Several years after that classic study, another study reported on the use of an anesthesia display, known as the integrated graphic anesthesia display (IGAD), that showed variables grouped by organ system, presented figures in color, employed simplified presentation techniques, and took advantage of principles of human factors, such as the principle of natural affordances by, for example, expanding a red rectangle in proportion to cardiac output with height corresponding to stroke volume and width corresponding to heart rate [23]. The IGAD was compared with a traditional display by simulating four critical incidents and measuring how fast two groups of five anesthesiologists could identify events. Again a complex screen-based simulator was used in a part-task setting. The IGAD was variably associated with better performance. The investigators pointed out the many specific limitations in performing display-comparison research, as well as artifacts of part-task simulation. The major purpose of such exercises may be to inform the design of more ecologically valid studies in full-scale and immersive simulations.

In other research, a group used a high-fidelity simulation environment to systematically test and study an intelligent system for monitoring and diagnosing postcardiac surgery patients in an intensive care unit [24]. The investigators suggested that knowledge-based systems must operate with incomplete models and thus require practical experimental validations. Their long-term objective was to show how a human–computer team might perform better than a human alone. In this study, the intelligent system was shown to perform well in six naturalistic, complex scenarios. Clinicians then participated in full-scale simulation scenarios similar to the ones scripted for the intelligent system, although the clinicians had many other physical tasks. For the purposes of the experiment, clinicians worked alone and not in teams. Suggestions were made as to where the intelligent system might support observed clinician performance, such as incorporating hidden data streams (eg, chest tube drainage) into an integrated monitor display, or providing clinicians with decision-making guidance in ambiguous and highly risky situations. Although interest in computer-based decision-support systems has continued to grow significantly for many clinical settings, they have not yet been validated in full-scale simulators.

Recently, a study of 20 anesthesiologists in a high-fidelity simulation environment compared the effectiveness of a new graphical cardiovascular display with that of a traditional monitor [25]. The graphical display was advanced for its use of shapes and colors that are pre-attentively processed, thus decreasing mental workload. Performance in the mock operating room was assessed by measuring the time it took to detect adverse events, make diagnoses, and provide care, and by measuring the deviation of vital signs from baseline. Time-coded videotapes were reviewed and rated. In the scenario with a radical prostatectomy and 1.5 L of blood loss, participants detected myocardial ischemia 2 minutes sooner than those using the traditional display, and were more likely to administer proper treatment earlier. There were no significant differences in performance between groups in the second scenario, a total hip replacement with a transfusion reaction. This groundbreaking study suffered from several limitations, including nonblinding of the reviewers to experimental or control conditions because of logistical issues, technical limitations because of physical artifacts of the simulation manikin, dependence on limited simulator physiological and pharmacological models for determining "patient" outcomes, and unanswered questions about alteration of behavior during a simulation despite subject claims of realism. The potential for relevance, transfer, and generalization of studies of this type is significant, especially with expected progress in improving full-scale simulation validity.

Record-keeping

Three studies have used full-scale simulation in anesthesia to investigate record-keeping performance and practices [26–28]. Methods improved over time with the addition of a requirement for contemporaneous record-keeping and of more realistic elements. Findings included frequent and occasionally gross inaccuracies in charted values compared with a gold standard (simulation monitor data) in all studies, and reduced accuracy during critical incidents and periods of high workload.

In the one large study of 124 participants, age, level of training, and years in practice were unrelated to the quality of manual record-keeping. Only half the subjects used a trending monitor function to support charting, and their records revealed similar inaccuracies to those who did not use computerized records to assist them. Patterns of "smoothing" physiological parameters were not commented on, yet this behavior has been well reported in studies of actual automated record-keeping in anesthesia. Although the investigators offered several hypotheses about the subjects' handling of "artifacts" when keeping records, no after-action reviews or debriefings were available to further understand these behaviors and "artifacts" were not defined. That is, it was never determined whether these were true artifacts or actual but extreme values. Research on automated record systems in actual clinical care has shown that they do not increase workload, but few such systems are in use.

The only other study found using simulation to study record-keeping practice concerned the management of a shoulder dystocia [29]. This study is mentioned because of its uniqueness, because of the paucity of work in this area, and because of the obvious interest of anesthesiology in obstetrical practice. The scenario made use of a birthing simulator, charts, and role players in a clinical setting. Obstetrical residents' delivery notes were collected to assess the presence and quality of 15 variables. Seventy-six percent recorded < 10 of the note components, only 18% charted which shoulder was anterior, and less than half estimated how long the head-to-body delivery interval lasted. Although the investigators mentioned that good record-keeping supports maintenance of situation awareness and thus improves care, their ultimate conclusion was flawed. Instead of aiming to better "train" residents to perfect post hoc event documentation as a primary strategy, efforts should have been directed toward analyzing task components and relationships as discussed previously. Sustained, successful remediation can only occur if the solution takes into account the tasks, tools, and human performance strengths and weaknesses as the units of analysis. Simulation can play a key role in the analysis and in adopting the best solutions.

Presumably, the ability to capture all values—real and artifactual, combined with the functionality to identify and comment on artifacts—may have a salutary effect on both practice and the ability to defend appropriate care when substandard care is claimed. It is also likely that the existence of a very large database of end-to-end accurate documentation for all cases will further support defense of cases with bad outcomes but no breach of standard of care, since physiological aberrations of significant degree will likely be found normative in many cases of good outcomes.

Other clinical tasks

Simulation has been applied to study performance in many different anesthesia tasks, including, for example, airway management and ventilation. These will not be discussed here for such a discussion would inherently emphasize performance assessments, training improvement, or limited task analyses. Theoretically, simulation could profitably be used to both study and possibly improve safety and efficiency of a wide range of selected activities, from blood transfusion in the exsanguinating patient to preventing wrong-site surgery in cases with high-risk factors for systems failures (eg, multiple surgeons, services, and procedures in the same patient; altered scheduling; transitions in care). Return on investment in complex and costly full-scale immersive simulations could be increased by conducting episodes-of-care simulations that incorporate many different tasks of interest for future analysis.

Adverse event analysis

Simulation has not been well appreciated for its use in understanding the causes, relationships, and evolution of specific adverse events. This topic could be discussed under systems applications as well, but these cases are mentioned here for their relatively narrow task focus. Admittedly, "stop rules" for guiding the bounds of adverse event investigation are by nature arbitrary [30], and it is important to keep in mind hidden, abstract, and latent organizational factors that set the stage for the occurrence of events downstream [31].

In 1995, one of the first widely noted cases of medical error—the death of previously healthy 7-year-old Ben Kolb from an accidental injection of concentrated adrenaline instead of lidocaine—helped catalyze the patient safety movement [32]. A painstaking re-creation of the ambulatory surgical operating room suite and simulation of the sequence thought to have taken place revealed many contributory hazard factors in the practices used to prepare and inject medications before beginning the surgery, processes that could be redesigned out of the task.

Formal and thorough operating room fire investigations typically use re-creations of the original scene in addition to experimental simulations to test theories about causality. In one government-sponsored investigation to better understand environmental conditions, a full-term mother was consented and draped for cesarean section. Prepping with swabs and solutions was then demonstrated. As part of the simulation, dozens of immediate, factors related to the local physical setting were taken into consideration [33]. In a case report from the anesthesia literature, a head-and-neck operating room fire was simulated in a detailed laboratory experiment using a full-scale manikin to recreate the circumstances of the fire [34]. The experiment was done nine times, four repeated to mimic the actual occurrence and five times to alter variables of interest to determine effect on outcome. An expert in medical adverse-event investigation contested the published conclusions in an exchange of letters with the investigators. That expert asserted, among other things, that the manikin wasn't warmed to body temperature, that the testing room did not have high ventilation turnover similar to that of an operating room, and that aluminum foil at the point of electrosurgical cautery was used instead of a more adequate substitute for human skin, such as pig skin [35,36]. In another operating room fire known to have a laser ignition source, a simulated re-creation in an actual reconstituted operating room suggested that the key factors in starting the fire were the surgeon's use of the foot pedal for laser operation, its mode of operation, and the typical location for this task.

The goal here is not to contest the validity of any conclusions about causality in these events, but to stress the very high reliance on fidelity and validity of the simulations, and the level of detail of task analysis required to make firm judgments. By contrast, typical immersive operating room simulations for training and most research do not strive for this level of validity, nor could they accomplish it because current pharmacological and physiological models are still emerging and the costs of full organizational fidelity would be prohibitive.

In a unique study using a simulated emergency pediatric department resuscitation setting, investigators studied the incidence of medication errors [37]. A manikin of unstated type represented the patient, and no details were given regarding the fidelity of defibrillation, airway management, or other procedures. However, actual drugs, syringes, intravenous equipment, needles, documentation, and other elements of medication administration were used, so that a high degree of ecological validity was attempted for the task of interest. Eight mock resuscitations were conducted on each of 35 subjects.

Despite three observers per case and professional videotapes of scenarios, it could not be determined in 17 instances whether or not the ordered drug was given. Post hoc chemical analyses were performed on the contents of 58 actual syringes. In four cases, deviation from the expected dose was at least 50%, and in nine syringes there was a deviation of <20%. A number of other performance failures occurred in medication administration. The simulation also demonstrated resilience to performance failure as four 10-fold overdoses were trapped before reaching the "patient." In essence, the investigators staged a simulated emergency, recorded data about performance, including unplanned adverse events, and used sophisticated techniques to investigate them with major implications for actual practice, morbidity, and mortality case reviews, and for systems improvement.

Devices

Simulation has long been a component of medical device design, usability studies, and training. The progressive development of full-scale, immersive simulation has now made it possible to more fully evaluate medical devices, and application studies are beginning to emerge. The U.S. Food and Drug Administration (FDA) has issued a document, Medical Device Use-Safety: Incorporating Human Factors Engineering into Risk Management, to guide industry and FDA premarket and design control reviewers [38]. Simulation can support many of the expected risk-management activities taken in device development. Simulation can be used, for example, (1) to identify and describe use scenarios resulting in hazards, including potentially those discovered from simulation "stress tests" as well as from simulated investigations of actual, reported near misses and adverse events; (2) to develop and verify mitigation and control strategies for use-related hazards; and (3) to determine if new hazards have been introduced.

The document emphasizes the importance of creating valid test scenarios and settings for usability testing.

> The unpredictability of human behavior, the complexity of medical device user interfaces, and the variability of use environments produce user-related hazards that can be difficult or impossible to identify or understand analytically.... *Empirical approaches* derive information from actual or simulated *use* of devices....they allow for previously *unanticipated use scenarios* resulting in hazards to be identified and described [38].

Critical, error-prone tasks and points where performance is most likely to fall short, as described above, can be both prospectively identified as well as captured descriptively through properly designed scenarios. In addition, characteristics of users involved in evaluation and testing must be carefully considered. Users of manufacturer-sponsored studies might be more biased, more capable, more motivated, or better informed than typical users. Also, in comparison with typical users, users of manufacturer-sponsored studies may have received more training. When device studies are embedded in full-scale simulations, users may also display more naturalistic behavior while multitasking as opposed to being allowed to focus simply on the device of interest.

Choice of available tools

One recent study used advanced simulation to investigate intraosseous vascular access in the treatment of chemical warfare casualties [39]. Because current protocols for emergency medical treatment of these patients assume no intravenous access, intramuscular access is assumed. However, poor perfusion in shock states may result in failure of intramuscular medical therapy. The investigators therefore studied a new, spring-driven, trigger-operated intraosseous device for adult and pediatric use by subjects who were also wearing bulky protective clothing and immersed in a high-fidelity bioterrorism simulation that included smoke, sirens, flashing lights, and manikins specially adapted to accept intraosseous placement. Scenarios were developed with expert assistance and based on data from reported casualties. Successful intraosseous cannulation was associated with faster simulated physiological uptake of antidote given the properties of noncollapsible marrow venous plexi. Length of treatment was significantly longer in the control group, and survival rate higher in the study group. Additional field data was gathered on hazardous use of the intraosseous apparatus and incorporated into training. A change in the treatment protocol for chemical warfare casualties was recommended.

In a case involving the selection of an emergency surgical airway kit, a trial on humans was felt to be unethical [40]. Four available kits were studied using a high-fidelity simulator during resuscitation scenarios with a scripted sense of urgency. Assessment criteria included ability to achieve a surgical airway, time to achieve oxygen pressure in arterial blood of 100 mm Hg, ease of fixation, trauma to surrounding structures, trauma to the kits, and overall subjective preference. Two sets had higher failure rates and complications, and one of the other two could be put in use faster, was preferred by most users, and consequently was incorporated into actual clinical operations.

Usability

Several key simulation-based usability studies are discussed. Reference to the complete methods and discussions is encouraged to better understand the limitations and nuances of advanced usability work, and to design additional studies that, by their nature, are quite context-dependent on device, setting, use, and user. Zhang and colleagues [41] describe for medical device usability studies an excellent framework that has not apparently been applied with advanced simulation methods [41]. To guide evaluation, Zhang and colleagues offer 14 Nielsen-Shierderman heuristics based on several prior systems. These include, for example, visibility of device system state, match between system and world, minimization of memory load, information feedback, flexibility, efficiency, quality of error messages, and reversible actions. Problems are also given a score on a severity rating scale from 0 (no problem) to 4 (usability catastrophe). The heuristics, initially developed to evaluate computer interfaces, were adapted for medical devices and could well inform simulation-based investigations of various human–machine systems.

As described in another study, a full-scale anesthesia simulation was employed for the first time to evaluate a prototype new drug administration system designed to reduce errors [42]. Because of the expected changes in workflow with attendant risks and possible unintended consequences, simulation trials, including performance stress tests, preceded introduction into actual practice. The new system included trays, color and bar-coded labeling of prefilled syringes, and automatic visual and auditory verification of syringes just before administration. The same subjects also compared the new system to the traditional method of drug administration. All 10 anesthetists felt the new system to be safer than the traditional system and of comparable usability. The new system reduced workload as assessed by subjects and observers, and provided much greater certainty that a certain drug (antibiotic) had indeed been administered instead of relying on memory or searching for empty ampoules. Sixty open-ended narrative comments by users in 10 categories helped to refine the new system.

Another investigation related to medication safety used a low-fidelity manikin in an actual clinical setting with resuscitation equipment, drugs, and associated devices [43]. Subjects conducted resuscitations in the conventional way in the control group. In the experimental group subjects conducted resuscitations with the decision aid of Broselow tape and color-coded materials. All scenarios were videotaped and coded. The study design was a two-treatment, two-period crossover trial with randomization of treatment. Evaluations measured deviation from recommended dosage ranges and levels of comfort with managing pediatric resuscitations. The intervention group made many fewer errors in drug dosing and made no large "sizing deviations" in judgments about proper endotracheal tubes, nasogastric catheters, and urinary catheters in this pediatric study. The results showed showed high usability and satisfaction with the Broselow tapes decision aid.

Like computer-based "glass cockpits" in aviation, anesthesia delivery systems are becoming more complex and opaque to clinicians. Typically,

training in the use of new systems is brief, is conducted by industry representatives, and occurs in actual clinical settings only to the degree that expert
users are present to answer questions during initial rollout on actual
patients. In one case, investigators took the novel step of conducting a randomized, controlled prospective trial involving the introduction of a Drager
Fabius GS anesthesia delivery system into actual practice [44]. Fifteen residents all received conventional training by company representatives, with
half receiving additional training through full-scale simulations. All were
then tested in complex full-scale simulated anesthetic crises using the new
system. Performance was assessed as also were design features that were
common sources of error. Because all the residents had extensive training
experience with the full simulation system, lack of familiarity during the trial
was not an issue. There was, however, no additional counterbalancing training time or method other than simulation offered to the control group. Residents who had received simulation training performed significantly better
than the control group. Also, residents who had received simulation training
made no errors with the equipment in the first scenario compared with 14
errors made by the control group. Confidence about usability before testing
in critical incident simulation scenarios was uniformly exaggerated by both
the simulator-trained and control groups, strongly suggesting that the introduction of new, complex equipment presents risks that practitioners
underestimate.

Advanced infusion pumps have introduced new types of injuries as well
as convenience and comfort. Peripheral and central intravenous, epidural,
wound, and implantable devices are commonplace. Some are controlled
by patients, with violations made by family and friends. Although "free
flow" has been designed out of current pump systems, and changes have
been made to reduce programming interface errors after a series of adverse
events and deaths, new hazards and additional complexity are continually
being introduced by adding new functionalities and cost-saving features
(eg, a single apparatus with one pump, a double cassette, and two intravenous solutions). No usability studies with these types of devices and full-
scale simulations were found. In the world of immersive simulation training,
however, complex infusion devices are often included to enrich management
challenges in scenarios and create human factor performance material for
post hoc debriefings. One elegant study on the usability of patient-controlled
analgesia devices used screen-based simulation to inform researchers who
might extend these methods to full-scale simulation [45].

Systems-level simulations

The complexity and cost of full-scale, immersive, systems-level simulations limits their application on a wide scale. Fifteen years of experience
with high-fidelity simulation in anesthesia and a decade in other disciplines

has now converged with a growing interest in systems thinking and the building of enough infrastructure to begin to develop this area. This article has suggested three physical representations defining systems-level simulations that mapped to the dimensions of complexity, scale, and organizational features. Fig. 2 illustrates how simulation methods might improve iterative systems.

Although discussion of computational simulation methods is beyond the scope of this article, such approaches lend themselves specifically to questions directed at the systems level because of the large number of elements and their interrelationships. Costs of running additional simulations are low, and models can be iteratively built and refined over time. Population-based simulation models of disease, patient flow, and resource management have grown more sophisticated. No studies were found that used a crosswalk between computational and physical representational full-scale simulations to increase ecological validity in either, but that time is not likely to be far away. Additional sources of data for systems simulations can be found in large public databases and in other reporting databases. These are useful for both gathering the necessary technical and historical details from actual cases and for identifying and focusing on patterns that reveal gaps and bottlenecks in systems. For example, the author reviewed over 200 reports of blood transfusion system incidents sent to the FDA and acquired through the Freedom of Information Act to inform the development of transfusion system simulations at the clinical end of operations with a blood bank interface.

In anesthesiology and perioperative care, appropriate settings for systems simulation could include multiple simultaneously interacting operating rooms with a control desk function, a recovery room with multiple patients, a postoperative intensive care unit, a preoperative clinic, a support statistical laboratory, or any combination of the above using manikins, standardized patient actors, consultants, telephones, pagers, and computer communications to minimize actual physical representational space. The unit of analysis in emergency medicine is more typically at the multipatient level, with emphasis on stabilization and disposition of individuals during constant workload fluctuations. In the first example of a multipatient small-systems simulation, three staggered patients were simulated with an interdisciplinary emergency department crew, a mix of computerized manikins and standard patients, and multiple simulation devices (eg, simulated mobile ultrasound equipment), with use of pass-through consultants and paramedics, and telephone and pager communications to simulate external information channels [17]. Other modalities could have included communication with actual state poison control offices and other resources.

One of the most extensive ongoing uses of systems-level simulations is underway with an idealized pediatric sedation service at an academic medical center [46]. A combination of simulation methods are used, including "crash dummy" or in situ tests of system function, simulations to aid task analysis, and full-scale training simulations. Simulations with the pediatric sedation service are also used to analyze events, perform observational studies, and test expert opinions.

In situ simulations are just beginning to grow more popular, although little information about such simulations has been published. A recent preliminary on-line report discusses the use of a mobile simulator to probe possible operational deficiencies in a newly built hospital emergency department just before occupancy [47]. Using scenarios involving cardiac arrest, multitrauma, uroseptic shock, and pediatric toxicology, the study uncovered remediable issues with unfavorable location of equipment, inadequate procedural surfaces, and insufficient personnel orientation. Another recent report from an aeromedical transport helicopter service affiliated with an emergency medicine residency training program described in situ training simulations in the actual helicopter running at flight-idle engine speeds on the ground [48]. This was more of a feasibility study in a unique clinical setting than a systems simulation because it did not appear that any care infrastructure was represented. Even so, it was well received and the model has the potential for including complex elements in pre-hospital and transition-to-hospital care. At least four recently funded projects in the first federal competition for health care simulation research will be using in situ methods to take advantage of actual systems infrastructure for research and training [49].

Interest in improving medical disaster management generally and response to terrorism specifically has resulted in large investments in multiple-manikin–type simulation exercises for civilian and military use. Much of the literature about such exercises appears to be descriptive, to be in the form of feasibility studies, or to be oriented for training. The first networked full-scale simulation system has been commercialized recently, enabling groups of simulation devices to be controlled from a central computer station, allowing multiple simultaneous levels of focus during a scenario, and providing for the electronic transfer of a manikin patient's physiological and pharmacological state to a distant manikin [50]. This technology will catalyze experimentation with physically simulated microsystems, health care organizations, and vertically and horizontally integrated medical disaster responses.

Summary

Medical simulation is maturing as a discipline and an industry. Organizational development of simulation centers and growth of interdisciplinary social research networks are continuing. Natural expansion of interest in simulation applications at the microsystem level of impact—the smallest replicable organizational unit—is occurring. Absent a major recession or war, the demand by external health care stakeholders for improved safety and quality will continue to positively influence these trends. Investigations of human factors using simulation will become more common as new technologies and procedures proliferate. Such investigations will also help define and improve simulation validity. One could make a case for ultimately institutionalizing simulation-based training for all new devices, procedures, and personnel. Lessons from other high-consequence industries have shown, however, that barriers to logistically complex, expensive simulations will remain. It will still be challenging to recruit expert and other subjects, perform studies with enough participants, understand and control confounding factors, and provide ecological validity. Future disruptive technologies may make some of these issues moot, however.

References

[1] Rall M, Gaba D. Patient simulators, vol. 2. In: Miller R, Fleisher L, Johns R, et al, editors. Miller's anesthesia. Philadelphia: Elsevier/Churchill Livingstone; 2005. p. 3073–103.

[2] Rall M, Gaba D. Human performance and patient safety, vol. 2. In: Miller R, Fleisher L, Johns R, et al, editors. Miller's anesthesia. Philadelphia: Elsevier/Churchill Livingstone; 2005. p. 3021–68.

[3] International Ergonomics Association (IEA). IEA Council definition of ergonomics adopted 2000. Available at: http://www.iea.cc/browse.php?contID=what_is_ergonomics. Accessed May 13, 2007.

[4] WordNet. Available at: http://wordnet.princeton.edu/perl/webwn?s=system&sub=Search+WordNet&o2=&o0=1&o7=&o5=&o1=1&o6=&o4=&o3=&h=. Accessed May 13, 2007.

[5] Nelson EC, Batalden PB, Mohr JJ, et al. Building a quality future. Front Health Serv Manage 1998;15:3–32.

[6] Small SD. Scenario design. In: Gaba D, Kurrek M, Small SD, editors. Instructors' manual for anesthesia crisis resource management. Toronto: The Working Group for Training in Anesthesia Crisis Resource Management; 1995. p. 69–85.

[7] Weinger M, Herndon O, Zornow M, et al. An objective methodology for task analysis and workload assessment in anesthesia providers. Anesthesiology 1994;80:77–92.

[8] Manser T, Wehner T. Analysing action sequences: variations in action density in the administration of anesthesia. Cognition Technology and Work 2002;4:71–81.

[9] Manser T, Rall M, Schaedle B, et al. Comparison of action density patterns between clinical and simulator settings. Eur J Anaesthesiol 2003;20:841A.

[10] Endsley M. Design and evaluation for situation awareness enhancement. Proc of the human factors society 32 Annual Meeting. Santa Monica (CA): Human Factors Society; 1988; 97–101.

[11] Gaba D, Howard S, Small S. Situation awareness in anesthesiology. Hum Factors 1995;37: 20–31.

[12] Wright M, Taekman J, Endsley M. Objective measures of situation awareness in a simulated medical environment. Qual Saf Health Care 2004;13(Suppl 1):65–71.

[13] Zhang Y, Drews F, Westenskow D, et al. Effect of integrated graphical displays on situation awareness in anesthesiology. Cognition Technology and Work 2002;4:82–90.

[14] Howard S, Gaba D, Smith B, et al. Simulation study of rested versus sleep-deprived anesthesiologists. Anesthesiology 2003;98(6):1345–55.

[15] Streufert S, Satish U. Graphic representations of processing structure: the time-event-matrix. J Appl Soc Psychol 1997;27:2122–48.

[16] Zsambok C. Naturalistic decision making: where are we now? In: Zsambok C, Klein G, editors. Naturalistic decision making. Mahwah (NJ): Lawrence Erlbaum Associates; 1997. p. 5.

[17] Small SD, Wuerz R, Simon R, et al. Demonstration of high fidelity simulation team training for emergency medicine. Acad Emerg Med 1999;6:312–23.
[18] Streufert S, Satish U, Gingrich D, et al. Excess coffee consumption in simulated complex work settings: detriment or facilitation of performance? J Appl Psychol 1997;82(5):774–82.
[19] Satish U, Streufert S, Dewan M, et al. Improvements in simulated real world relevant performance for patients with seasonal allergic rhinitis: impact of desloratadine. Allergy 2004;59:415–20.
[20] Streufert S, DePadova A, McGlynn T, et al. Impact of beta-blockade on complex cognitive functioning. Am Heart J 1988;11:311–8.
[21] Satish U, Streufert S, Marshall R, et al. Strategic management simulation as a novel way to measure resident competencies. Am J Surg 2001;181:557–61.
[22] Gurushanthaiah K, Weinger MB, Englund CE. Visual display format affects the ability of anesthesiologists to detect acute physiologic changes. A laboratory study employing a clinical display simulator. Anesthesiology 1995;83:1184–93.
[23] Michels P, Gravenstein D, Westenskow DR. An integrated graphic data display improves detection and identification of critical events during anesthesia. J Clin Monit 1997;13:249–59.
[24] Larsson JE, Hayes-Roth B, Gaba DM, et al. Evaluation of a medical diagnosis system using simulator test scenarios. Artif Intell Med 1997;11:119–40.
[25] Agutter J, Drews F, Syroid N, et al. Evaluation of graphic cardiovascular display in a high-fidelity simulator. Anesth Analg 2003;97:1403–13.
[26] Byrne AJ, Sellen AJ, Jones JG. Errors on anaesthetic record charts as a measure of anaesthetic performance during simulated critical incidents. Br J Anaesth 1998;80:58–62.
[27] Devitt JH, Rapanos T, Kurrek M, et al. The anesthetic record: accuracy and completeness. Can J Anaesth 1999;46:122–8.
[28] Byrne AJ, Jones JG. Inaccurate reporting of simulated critical anaesthetic incidents. Br J Anaesth 1997;78:637–41.
[29] Deering S, Poggi S, Hodor J, et al. Evaluation of residents' delivery notes after a simulated shoulder dystocia. Obstet Gynecol 2004;104:667–70.
[30] Rasmussen J. The role of error in organizing behavior. Ergonomics 1990;33:1185–90.
[31] Reason J. Managing the risks of organizational accidents. London: Ashgate; 1997.
[32] Belkin L. How can we save the next victim? The New York Times. June 15, 1997.
[33] Accidental fire causing serious harm to a patient during surgery in an operating theatre. Fire Investigation Report, New Zealand Fire Service, Waitakere City Fire District, Fire incident ICAD No.A319786.
[34] Barker S, Polson S. Fire in the operating room: a case report and laboratory study. Anesth Analg 2001;93(4):960–5.
[35] Bruley M, de Richemond A. Supplemental oxygen versus latent alcohol vapors as surgical fire precursors. Lett. Ed. Anesth Analg 2002;95:1464.
[36] Barker S. Reply—supplemental oxygen versus latent alcohol vapors as surgical fire precursors. Lett. Ed. Anesth Analg 2002;95:1464–5.
[37] Kozer E, Seto W, Verjee Z, et al. Prospective observational study on the incidence of medication errors during simulated resuscitation in a paediatric emergency department. BMJ 2004;329:1321.
[38] Kaye R, Crowley J. Guidance for industry and FDA premarket and design control reviews. Medical device use-safety: incorporating human factors engineering into risk management. Document issued on July 18, 2000, U.S. Department of health and human services, food and drug administration center for devices and radiological health, division of device user programs and systems analysis, office of health and industry programs. Available at: http://www.fda.gov/cdrh/humfac/1497.html. Accessed May 13, 2007.
[39] Vardi A, Berkenstadt H, Levin I, et al. Intraosseous vascular access in the treatment of chemical warfare casualties assessed by advanced simulation: proposed alteration of treatment protocol. Anesth Analg 2004;98:1753–8.

[40] Vadodaria B, Gandhi S, McIndoe A. Selection of an emergency cricothyroidotomy kit for clinical use by dynamic evaluation on a (METI) human patient simulator, International Meeting on Medical Simulation. San Diego (CA): Society for Medical Stimulation; 2003.

[41] Zhang J, Johnson T, Patel V, et al. Using usability heuristics to evaluate patient safety of medical devices. J Biomed Inform 2003;36:23–30.

[42] Merry AF, Webster CS, Weller J, et al. Evaluation in an anaesthetic simulator of a prototype of a new drug administration system designed to reduce error. Anaesthesia 2002;57:256–63.

[43] Shah A, Frush K, Luo X, et al. Effect of an intervention standardization system on pediatric dosing and equipment size determination. Arch Pediatr Adolesc Med 2003;157:229–36.

[44] Dalley P, Robinson B, Weller J, et al. The use of high-fidelity human patient simulation and the introduction of new anesthesia delivery systems. Anesth Analg 2004;99:1737–41.

[45] Lin L, Isla R, Doniz K, et al. Applying human factors to the design of medical equipment: patient-controlled analgesia. J Clin Monit Comput 1998;14:253–63.

[46] Blike G, Cravero J, Nelson E. Same patients, same critical events—different systems of care, different outcomes: description of a human factors approach aimed at improving the efficacy and safety of sedation/analgesia care. Qual Manag Health Care 2001;10(1):17–36.

[47] Kobayashi L, Shapiro M, Sucov A, et al. Portable advanced medical simulation for new emergency department testing and orientation. Acad Emerg Med 2006; published online before print April 24. doi:10.1197/j.aem.2006.01.023.

[48] Wright S, Lindsell C, Hinckley W, et al. High fidelity medical simulation in the difficult environment of a helicopter: feasibility, self-efficacy and cost. BMC Med Educ 2006;6:49. Published online 2006 October 5. doi:10.1186/1472-6920-6-49.

[49] Agency for Healthcare Research and Quality. Improving patient safety through simulation research. Available at: http://www.ahrq.gov/qual/simulproj.htm. Accessed May 13, 2007.

[50] Medical Education Technologies, Inc. Available at: http://www.meti.com/Product_METI_LiVE.html. Accessed May 13, 2007.

ANESTHESIOLOGY
CLINICS

ELSEVIER
SAUNDERS
Anesthesiology Clin
25 (2007) 261–269

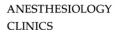

Credentialing and Certifying with Simulation

Amitai Ziv, MD, MHA[a,b,*], Orit Rubin, PhD[a,c],
Avner Sidi, MD,[b,d,e], Haim Berkenstadt, MD[a,b,d]

[a]The Israel Center for Medical Simulation (MSR), Chaim Sheba Medical Center,
Tel-Hashomer 52621, Israel
[b]Tel Aviv University Sackler School of Medicine, Jerusalem, Israel
[c]The National Institute for Testing and Evaluation, Jerusalem, Israel
[d]The Israeli Board Examination Committee in Anesthesiology, Jerusalem, Israel
[e]Department of Anesthesiology and Intensive Care, Chaim Sheba Medical Center,
Tel-Hashomer 52621, Israel

Assessment and evaluation are an integral part of any educational and training process, and it is human nature that students at all levels of training respond by studying more seriously for the parts of the course or training that are assessed. To promote and enhance effective learning successfully, simulation and other teaching methods should be both formative and summative, because the ultimate goal is to ensure professional competence [1]. The latter was defined by Epstein and Hundert [2] as the "habitual and judicious use of communication, knowledge, technical skills, clinical reasoning, emotions, values, and reflection in daily practice for the benefit of the individual and community being served." This article describes a model of medical competence, and focuses on the use of medical simulation in assessment and evaluation of different levels of clinical competence using examples from experience.

Miller's model of medical competence

A well-established model of medical competence was suggested by Miller [3]. Miller's pyramid presents four layers of competence, defined as (1) knows, (2) knows how, (3) shows how, and (4) does.

* Corresponding author. The Israel Center for Medical Simulation (MSR), Chaim Sheba Medical Center, Tel-Hashomer 52621, Israel.
   E-mail address: amitai.ziv@sheba.health.gov.il (A. Ziv).

1932-2275/07/$ - see front matter © 2007 Elsevier Inc. All rights reserved.
doi:10.1016/j.anclin.2007.03.002   *anesthesiology.theclinics.com*

1. The "knows" level refers to the recall of facts, principles, and theories. The traditional method of assessing this level was the essay, replaced later by multiple-choice tests, to assess the recall and application of knowledge [4].

2. The "knows how" level involves the ability to solve problems and describe procedures. Paper- or computer-based simulations are involved in the assessment of this layer, replacing gradually the traditional clinical and oral examinations that suffer from low correlations, insufficient agreement between examiners, and low reliability [5]. An example for such a test that can be used in both written [6] and computer-based form [7] is the presentation of a short description of a clinical scenario in which a problem is presented followed by a number of multiple-choice questions or short answer open-ended questions referring for essential decisions [8]. Another format is the extended-matching question [9], where the examinee needs to match the most appropriate response from one list to another list of related cases.

3. At the "shows how" level of medical competence examinees need to demonstrate their clinical performance. The introduction of objective structured clinical examination in the 1970s was the breakthrough in clinical testing at this level [10]. This topic is presented in more detail later in this article, and examples for objective structured clinical examination and simulation-based assessment and evaluation are provided.

4. The "does" level, representing the top layer of Miller's pyramid, involves testing of clinical performance in the working environment using such techniques as clinical work sampling [11], practice video recording [12], peers rating [13], and simulated patients–based examinations [14]. The Royal College of General Practitioners developed a final professional licensing examination in which candidates for certification present several best-case videotapes of their performance in real clinical settings to a trained examiner who uses specified criteria for evaluation [15].

Objective structured clinical examination

The objective structures clinical examination (OSCE) consists of multiple stations around which examinees rotate and perform and are assessed on specific tasks by examiners or by simulated patients on whom the task was performed [16]. OSCE is widely used for assessment and certification around the world. This tool is used for evaluation of foreign doctors wishing to practice in the United States [17]; the General Medical Council [18]; the Medical Council of Canada [19]; and for the evaluation of graduates of medical schools [20], residents in pediatrics [21], surgery [22], and dentists [23]. Recently, the National Board of Medical Examiners in the United States has introduced the simulation-based clinical skills examination to all graduates of medical school in the United States [24], reflecting a major shift in the field of medical

accreditation and licensure toward acknowledging the crucial role of performance assessment as an important component of professional accreditation.

The incorporation of medical simulation to OSCE-based evaluation allows
the assessment of clinical and task-based performance and increases the au-
thenticity of the assessment method. Simulation based assessment in anesthesia has been explored and studied since the introduction of the high-fidelity
anesthesia simulators in the early 1990s. This new generation of simulators
opened the horizons of medical educators in anesthesia because it provided
a structured and standardized platform for training and assessment in this
field [25]. Indeed, some studies assessed the interrater reliability [26] and construct validity [27,28] of high-fidelity medical simulation in anesthesia, and
a multi-institutional study validated simulation-based scenarios as a tool
for residents' evaluation [29]. In other institutions simulation is being used
as a practical tool for evaluation and even accreditation. The New York State
Society of Anesthesiologists reported the use of a human patient simulator in
the evaluation and development of a remedial prescription for an anesthesiologist with lapsed medical skills [30]. In the university hospital in Heidelberg,
full-scale simulation was used for accreditation of anesthesia nurses [31]; in
the department of anesthesiology in Rochester the human patient simulator
was reported to be used to credential first-year anesthesiology residents for
taking overnight call [32]; and a mandatory competency-based difficult airway
management training is performed at the University of Pittsburgh department
of anesthesiology [33].

In Israel, the Israel Center for Medical Simulation (MSR) [34] is involved
in three unique high-stakes simulation-based accreditation projects: (1) medical school candidates' selection, (2) national board examination in anesthesiology, and (3) national accreditation for paramedics. MSR also takes part
in a national mandatory course for interns and in other courses involving
performance assessment of military and civilian medical team in the pre-
and in-hospital environments. Two of these projects are described for
more comprehensive understanding of the processes involved in incorporating simulation for assessment and accreditation.

Admission to Tel Aviv University Sackler School of Medicine

Most medical schools' selection processes rely mainly on tools that measure cognitive factors. The most common tools record candidates' previous
academic achievements, coupled with norm-referenced cognitive examinations [35]. These tools can be efficiently administered to large numbers of
candidates, produce data that can be objectively scored and analyzed, and
they are good predictors of students' academic success in medical school
[36]. Interviews incorporated to the admission process are the most com-
monly used tool for gaining insight into candidates' personal characteristics
[37], most of them used as disqualifying tools. Although the interview's face

validity is strong, interviewer biases and context biases have been shown to influence the results of the interview [38].

Recently, an OSCE-like exercise consisting of multiple mini-interviews was introduced by McMaster University in Canada [35]. In each encounter, a different type of interview-behavioral simulation was performed (eg, discussion of ethical dilemma, discussion of candidates' life history, or observation on candidates' communication with anxious patient). In Tel Aviv University Sackler School of Medicine an assessment center, similar to assessment centers customarily used in psychology and aviation, was initiated 3 years ago in cooperation with the MSR and the National Institute for Testing and Evaluation [39]. The center applies simulation as a central component of the assessment process, recognizing that interviews, questionnaires, and tests in which candidates verbally describe their behavior, tendencies, and so forth should be complemented by simulation-based assessment that allows direct observation of candidates' behaviors. Based on this rationale, and following a judgment and decision-making questionnaire and a biographic questionnaire, the behavioral assessment of candidates consists of six individual (OSCE-like) stations (6–9 minutes each) and two group stations (30 minutes each). Three of the simulation stations represent challenging humane encounters between an individual candidate and a simulated patient (role-playing actor) within a medical or nonmedical context, two debriefing stations for two of the simulations where the candidate is interviewed by a rater who had observed his or her behavior in one of the simulation stations, and one standardized personal interview station where candidates are interviewed on their attitudes toward the medical profession and about current medical issues. In each of the two group stations, a group of six candidates is asked to perform a task together. In the different stations candidates' behavior is observed and scored by trained faculty members using a structured assessment form. This form consists of four dimensions of personal characteristics: (1) interpersonal communication skills, (2) stress handling, (3) initiative and responsibility, and (4) self-awareness. According to the experiences gained in the years 2004 and 2005, the candidates and raters perceived the assessment center as a highly fair screening tool, and the new screening process resulted in an 18% to 20% change in the make-up of the accepted students each year (A. Ziv and O. Rubin, personal communication, 2006). Ongoing research is looking at the validity of this revolutionary assessment approach through prospective follow-up and assessment of the students as they continue their medical training.

The Israeli board examination in anesthesiology

Many institutions introduced the use of high-fidelity medical simulation into residents' training. The interrater reliability, construct validity, and value of simulation-based scenarios as an effective tool for the evaluation of residents have been explored. In the United Kingdom, OSCE was incorporated into the Fellow Royal College of Anesthesiologists (FRCA) examinations. The areas tested in the OSCE stations include resuscitation, technical skills, anatomy, history-taking, physical examination, communication skills, data interpretation, monitoring and measurement, anesthetic hazards, and statistics [40].

Acknowledging the fact that the Israeli board examination in anesthesiology lacked a performance evaluation component, and that this domain had not been a substantial part of training programs in the country, the Israeli Board of Anesthesiology Examination Committee decided 4 years ago to explore the potential of adding an OSCE component to the Board Examination process [41]. Following a process involving members of the Israeli Board of Anesthesiology Examination Committee, experts from the MSR and from Israel's National Institute for Testing and Evaluation, clinical conditions that anesthesiologists are required to handle competently and tasks pertaining to each of the conditions were defined. Tasks were then incorporated into hands-on simulation-based examination stations in the OSCE format. Stations include the following:

1. Trauma management: An emergency room environment and Sim-Man (Laerdal, Stavenger, Norway) simulator are used and examinees are expected to evaluate and treat a trauma casualty according to advanced trauma life support guidelines.
2. Resuscitation: As in the trauma station, using a Sim-Man (Laerdal, Stavenger, Norway) simulator, examinees are expected to evaluate and treat a patient according to advanced cardiac life-support guidelines.
3. Operating room crisis management: A full-scale simulated operating room and the High Fidelity Patient Simulator (METI, Gainesville, Florida) are used. In this scenario, examinees are called into the operating room to help a junior resident encountering a problem during anesthesia (eg, hypertension following the induction of general anesthesia).
4. Mechanical ventilation: Using a ventilator and an artificial lung, the examinees are asked to adjust the mechanical ventilation in response to changes in lung compliance or the results of arterial blood gases. (In the Israeli medical system these tasks are performed by physicians and not by respiratory therapists).
5. Regional anesthesia: Using a standardized-simulated patient (a role-playing actor) the examinee has to demonstrate familiarity with the relevant surface anatomy, place of needle insertion, needle direction, and amount of local anesthetics injected while performing regional anesthesia block. Complications induced by the procedure, including convulsions and pain during the injection of local anesthetics, are also demonstrated by the actor.

The process of examination included also the development of the assessment tools, orientation for the examinees, and preparation of examiners. The examination has been administered seven times in the past 4 years, and has gradually progressed from being a minor part of the oral board examination to a prerequisite component of this test.

The psychometric characteristics of this unique evaluation process and the candidates' perception of it were evaluated through exploring the following aspects: satisfaction and realism, interrater and intercase reliability, content validity and convergent validity, and error reduction [42]. The satisfaction according to a subjective feedback questionnaire was high (70%–90%), as was the realism (80%–90%). Scenarios used for the same clinical conditions had similar levels of difficulty. The rate of incongruence between examiners was low ($<15\%$). The mean interrater correlations were 0.89 to 0.76. The intercase reliability (internal consistency) correlations were calculated between the five OSCE stations' scores and were significant ($P<.01$) only between trauma and ventilation, and between resuscitation and regional and resuscitation and operating room crisis. The criterion-related or convergent validity correlation between the OSCE examination scores and the success rate at eight different clinical domains of the oral board examination did not reach statistical significance. The simulator effect on error reduction was evaluated and found effective. All major errors that were identified in the initial two examination periods disappeared in the next two periods.

Keys for success in incorporating simulation and objective structured clinical examination into assessment and evaluation

The incorporation of OSCE into the assessment of medical personnel involves a structured process of examination development, including the definition of assessment conditions, tasks, and scenarios on the basis of accepted medical protocols and broad professional consensus. This process contributes to the objectivity and the content and face validity of the examination, and also its positive reception by the medical community. According to the authors' experience, a major key for success in such a process is the cooperation between clinicians, experts in testing and evaluation, and experts in medical simulation. Parameters like interrater and intercase reliability, content and face validity, global rating and checklist rating, and pass-failed criteria are usually not familiar to clinicians, and assistance from experts in testing and evaluation is mandatory. Another key for success is to perform changes slowly and gradually to overcome opposition and fear from both examiners and examinees. That is the reason why the process of incorporating OSCE to the Israeli Boards in Anesthesiology is not finished, and parameters like preoperative evaluation and communication skills are not yet assessed.

In the process of adapting OSCE and simulation for testing and evaluation, one needs to remember that OSCE is best suited to testing clinical, technical, and practical skills and can do so across a very broad range.

Some aspects of clinical competence, like behavioral aspects, are probably better evaluated by the use of multiple ratings collected over a period of time during clinical work. Moreover, the OSCE is an expensive tool, and the testing of formal knowledge can be more cost effectively tested with written formats.

The availability of high-fidelity simulators in anesthesia and the well established OSCE model for performance assessment provide a unique opportunity. There is no doubt that incorporating simulation and OSCE for testing and evaluation should play a formative (training) and a summative (testing) role, involving the anesthesiology board, anesthesia departments, the participating examiners, and the examinees. The examination development process induced a critical appraisal of the current training and assessment paradigm, and led to exploration, definition, and prioritization of the critical clinical skills expected from a residency graduate. The examination also provided a rare glimpse at the authentic products of Israeli residencies, highlighting areas of strengths and weaknesses that could serve as guidelines to future modifications in the residency curriculum and practice.

References

[1] Wass V, Van der Vleuten C, Shatzer J, et al. Assessment of clinical competence. Lancet 2001; 357:945–9.
[2] Epstein RM, Hundert EM. Defining and assessing professional competence. JAMA 2002; 287:226–35.
[3] Miller GE. The assessment of clinical skills/competence/performance. Acad Med 1990;65: S63–7.
[4] Newble D. Techniques for measuring clinical competence: objective structured clinical examinations. Med Educ 2004;38:199–204.
[5] Hubbard JP. Measuring medical education. Philadelpia: Lea & Febiger; 1971.
[6] Page G, Bordage G. The medical council of Canada's key features project: a more valid written examination of clinical decision-making skills. Acad Med 1995;70:104–10.
[7] Schuwirth LWT. An approach to the assessment of medical problem solving: computerized case-based testing [dissertation]. . Netherlands: Universiteit Maastricht; 1998.
[8] Bordage G. An alternative approach to PMP's: the 'key-features' concept. In: Harden R, editor. Further developments in assessing clinical competence. Proceedings of the Second Ottawa Conference. Montreal (Canada): Can-Heal Publications; 1987. p. 59–75.
[9] Case SM, Swanson DB. Extended-matching items: a practical alternative to free response questions. Teach Learn Med 1993;5:107–15.
[10] Harden RM, Gleeson FA. Assessment of clinical competence using an objective structured clinical examination (OSCE). Med Educ 1979;13:41–54.
[11] Turnbull J, MacFadyen J, Van-Barneveld C, et al. Clinical work sampling: a new approach to the problem of in-training evaluation. J Gen Intern Med 2000;15:556–61.
[12] Ram P, Grol R, Rethans JJ, et al. Assessment of general practitioners by video observation of communicative and medical performance in daily practice: issues of validity, reliability and feasibility. Med Educ 1999;33:447–54.
[13] Ramsey PG, Wenrich MD, Carline JD, et al. Use of peer rating in physician performance. JAMA 1993;269:1655–60.
[14] Rethans J, Sturmans F, Drop M, et al. Assessment of performance in actual practice of general practitioners by use of standardized patients. Br J Gen Pract 1991;41:97–9.

[15] Lockie C. The examination for membership in the Royal College of General Practitioners of England. Royal College of General Practitioners 1990. Occasional Paper 46.

[16] Petrusa ER. Clinical performance assessment. In: Norman GR, Van der Vleuten CPM, Newble DI, editors. International handbook of research in medical education. Dordrecht: Kluwer Academic Publications; 2002.

[17] Ziv A, Ben-David MF, Sutnick AI, et al. Lessons learned from six years of international administrations of the ECFMG's SP-based clinical skills assessment. Acad Med 1998;73:84–91.

[18] Tombeson P, Fox RA, Dacre JA. Defining the content for the objective structured clinical examination component of the Professional and Linguistic Assessment Board examination: development of a blueprint. Med Educ 2000;34:566–72.

[19] Reznick RK, Blackmore D, Cohen R, et al. An objective structured clinical examination for the licentiate: report of the Medical Council of Canada: from research to reality. Acad Med 1992;67:487–94.

[20] Probert CS, Cahill DJ, McCann GL, et al. Traditional finals and OSCEs in predicting consultant and self-reported clinical skills of PRHOs: a pilot study. Med Educ 2003;37:597–602.

[21] Matsell DG, Wolfish NM, Hsu E. Reliability and validity of the objective structured clinical examination in paediatrics. Med Educ 1991;25(4):293–9.

[22] Schwartz RW, Witzke DB, Donnelly MB, et al. Assessing residents' clinical performance: cumulative results of a four-year study with the objective structured clinical examination. Surgery 1998;124:307–12.

[23] Boyd MA, Gerrow JD, Duquette P. Rethinking the OSCE as a tool for national competency evaluation. Eur J Dent Educ 2004;8(2):95.

[24] Papadakis MA. The step 2 clinical skills examination. N Engl J Med 2004;350:1703–5.

[25] Cooper JB, Taqueti VR. A brief history of the development of mannequin simulators for clinical education and training. Qual Saf Health Care 2004;13(Suppl 1):i11–8.

[26] Weller JM, Bloch M, Young S, et al. Evaluation of high fidelity patient simulator in assessment of performance of anaesthetists. Br J Anaesth 2003;90:43–7.

[27] Forrest FC, Taylor MA, Postlethwaite K, et al. Use of a high-fidelity simulator to develop testing of the technical performance of novice anaesthetists. Br J Anaesth 2002;88:338–44.

[28] Devitt JH, Kurrek MM, Cohen MM, et al. Testing internal consistency and construct validity during evaluation of performance in a patient simulator. Anesth Analg 1998;86:1160–4.

[29] Schwid HA, Rooke GA, Carline J, et al. Anesthesia Simulator Research Consortium. Evaluation of anesthesia residents using mannequin-based simulation: a multiinstitutional study. Anesthesiology 2002;97:1434–44.

[30] Rosenblatt MA, Abrams KJ, New York State Society of Anesthesiologists; Committee on Continuing Medical Education and Remediation; Remediation Sub-Committee. The use of a human patient simulator in the evaluation of and development of a remedial prescription for an anesthesiologist with lapsed medical skills. Anesth Analg 2002;94:149–53.

[31] Grube C, Sinner B, Boeker T, et al. The patient simulator for taking examinations: a cost effective tool? Anesthesiology 2001;95:A1202.

[32] Henson LC, Richardson MG, Stern DH, et al. Using human patient simulator to credential first year anesthesiology residents for taking overnight call. Presented as an abstract at the 2nd Annual International Meeting on Medical Simulation. Santa Fe (NM), January 14–18, 2002.

[33] Schaefer JJ. Mandatory competency-based difficult airway management training at the University of Pittsburgh Department of Anesthesiology. Presented as an abstract at the 4th Annual International Meeting on Medical Simulation. Santa Fe (NM), January 14–18, 2004.

[34] MSR Israel Center for Medical Simulation. Available at: http://www.msr.org.il/. Accessed October 2006.

[35] Eva KW, Reiter IH, Rosenfeld J, et al. The ability of the multiple mini-interview to predict preclerkship performance in medical school. Acad Med 2004;79:40–2.

[36] Spychalski AC, Quinones MA, Gaugler BB, et al. A survey of assessment center practices in organizations in the United States. Personnel Psychology 1997;50:71–90.

[37] Arthur W, Day EA, McNelly TL, et al. A meta-analysis of the criterion-related validity of assessment center dimensions. Personnel Psychology 2003;56:125–54.
[38] Lievens F. Assessor training strategies and their effects on accuracy, interrater reliability and discriminant validity. J Appl Psychol 2001;86:255–64.
[39] National Institute for Testing and Evaluation. Available at: http://www.nite.org.il/. Accessed October 2006.
[40] Anesthesia UK. Available at: http://www.frca.co.uk/SectionContents.aspx?sectionid=74. Accessed October 2006.
[41] Berkenstadt H, Ziv A, Gafni N, et al. Incorporating simulation-based objective structured clinical examination (OSCE) into the Israeli national board examination in anesthesiology. Anesth Analg 2006;102:853–8.
[42] Berkenstadt H, Ziv A, Gafni N, et al. The validation process of incorporating simulation-based accreditation into the anesthesiology Israeli national board exams. IMAJ 2006;10(8):728–33.

ANESTHESIOLOGY
CLINICS

ELSEVIER
SAUNDERS

Anesthesiology Clin
25 (2007) 271–282

Statewide Simulation Systems: The Next Step for Anesthesiology?

Michael Seropian, MD, FRCPC[a,b,c,f,*],
Dawn Dillman, MD[a], David Farris, MD[d,e]

[a]Department of Anesthesiology and Perioperative Medicine, Oregon Health & Science
University, 3181 SW Sam Jackson Park Road, MC UHS2, Portland, OR 97239, USA
[b]OHSU Simulation Center, 3181 SW Sam Jackson Park Road,
MC UHS2, Portland, OR 97239, USA
[c]Society for Simulation in Healthcare, ADP Plaza suite 100,
2525 First Avenue, Portland, OR 97201, USA
[d]Legacy Emanuel Hospital, Legacy Health System, Society for Simulation in Healthcare,
PMB 300 223 N. Guadalupe, Santa Fe, NM 87501, USA
[e]Emanuel Children's Hospital, 2801 N Gantenbein Avenue, Portland, OR 97227, USA
[f]Oregon Simulation Alliance, Oregon, USA

The Joint Commission on Accreditation of Health Care Organizations reported in 2002 that new graduates of American residencies and medical schools are ill-prepared to respond to crisis situations, to supervise care provided by others, and to perform complex skills [1]. The commission noted that health education continues to occur in "silos" at a time when nurses, physicians, pharmacists and allied health professionals must collaborate rather than just simply coexist. Numerous national studies have demonstrated that today's educational system does not provide students with the knowledge and skills necessary to lead and interact safely and effectively within a care-giving team. The Institute of Medicine (IOM) has issued several reports that have inspired an intense national dialog on patient safety and quality of care [2]. The IOM argues that interdisciplinary training should be a top priority in preparing the workforce to practice safely and effectively in today's health care environment. Simulation is specifically identified as a resource to address these issues.

* Corresponding author. Department of Anesthesiology and Perioperative Medicine, Oregon Health & Science University, 3181 SW Sam Jackson Park Road, MC UHS2, Portland, OR 97239.

E-mail address: seropian@ohsu.edu (M. Seropian).

Simulation is an educational methodology intended to provide learning exercises by closely mimicking practical, "real life" situations. Cockpit simulators in aviation and similar setups in the military have become invaluable training tools. Manikin-based simulation was introduced into health care 15 years ago but was initially very expensive, with a cost of $150,000 per simulator. Simulation technology today is much more affordable, ranging from $28,000 to $40,000 per simulator.

Simulation activities range from low-fidelity skill training, such as practicing injections on a training arm, to high-fidelity training sessions on sophisticated virtual reality skill trainers (eg, ultrasound and laparoscopic trainers), to interdisciplinary management of cardiac arrest in "real time" using sophisticated manikins with controllable responses. State-of-the-art simulation allows students and practitioners to learn by self-assessment and peer assessment in a safe, nonthreatening environment.

Beyond the obvious development of the knowledge base required for management of specific cases, health care simulation provides an opportunity to teach individuals from multiple disciplines simultaneously, which is basic to advanced cognitive and procedural knowledge. Skills in communication, professionalism, resource management, systems-based thinking, clinical judgment, and interdisciplinary team function can all be effectively taught. Nursing and allied health share with medicine the desire to augment discipline-specific curricula with interdisciplinary learning. Simulation provides an ideal venue.

Models for building capacity

Simulation education is becoming more pervasive with each passing month. Despite this, few standards exist for implementation, methods, and qualifications necessary to provide quality courses [3–5]. Only a few, mainly academic, institutions have the capabilities to formulate such standards. The need to leverage such expertise is more pressing than ever. In 2004, the American Society of Anesthesiologists (ASA) convened a workgroup on simulation education. Over the last 2 years, this group produced a white paper that discusses the criteria for a successful simulation program, as well as options for program certification that the ASA may want to consider [6]. While this work is important, progress will be difficult and slow without a distribution network for expertise in simulation.

This is where large-scale and, more specifically, statewide simulation networks become relevant. Such networks afford not only the possibility of meeting capacity needs for anesthesiologists, but also provide a venue for training trainers, setting standards, and bringing academic and nonacademic practices together. Furthermore, a statewide network that is appropriately designed opens the door to interdisciplinary activity. Interdisciplinary simulation has been problematic in the United States for a variety of reasons, such as difficulties related to traditional discipline silos, scheduling, and cost.

Statewide efforts are indeed underway in many states, including California, Colorado, Florida, Idaho, Michigan, Oregon, Pennsylvania, South Carolina, and Washington. Most of these collaboratives are limited in scope to either specific disciplines or sectors. Nursing is dominant in this approach. This is not surprising, as the use of simulation in nursing is far more common than it is in medicine. This, of course, will change as medicine adopts simulation and requests multiply for increased training opportunities.

There are current attempts in South Carolina and Washington to implement models across disciplines. These projects are in their early stages. Certain states have made statewide attempts at organizing for specific purposes. For instance, in New Jersey, the state's Department of Health and Senior Services has created a statewide program for education in disaster readiness that is meant to train providers across disciplines in mass casualty events. This program uses high-fidelity patient simulators in its curriculum to improve the depth of the educational experience for providers. However, there is no attempt to organize existing simulation resources for other purposes; simulation is limited to education for disaster readiness [7].

The Oregon experience—a statewide market-based approach

Oregon is the first state to implement simulation education across disciplines throughout the state. The model provides an example of how simulation can be successfully applied across a large and diverse area. This effort began in November 2003 and has expanded from one major center to programs at 23+ locations as of March 2007. The implementation strategy involved a phased build-up that gave the most importance to nursing in the early stages, with shifting emphasis in later stages to medicine and allied health. That shift is now occurring. By taking a major role in the collaboration, anesthesiologists are helping to guide implementation in an endeavor that may become a model for other groups in other states.

Advantages of a statewide system

A statewide simulation system has some obvious benefits and includes a variety of components and advantages:

- Multiple sites. A statewide simulation system, by providing several access points, can be more easily available to providers. For instance, a provider may be more likely to use a nearby resource for maintenance of certification activities because getting there takes less time from clinical productivity. In addition, by having multiple sites, different sites can sub-specialize and invest to become better equipped for certain types of simulation (eg, disaster readiness and obstetric emergencies).
- Communications network. In a statewide simulation system, the multiple sites communicate among one another, facilitating sharing of

intellectual resources, such as curriculum and problem-solving expertise, and physical resources.

- Audio-visual infrastructure and network for distance learning and sharing. A statewide simulation system can establish an audio-visual infrastructure and network for distance learning and sharing. This may be especially valuable for providers in rural or remote locations. Through an advanced telecommunications network, such providers can share valuable experiences, such as debriefing discussions, in real time.
- Closer relationships among content experts. By fostering relationships among content experts throughout a state, statewide networks may facilitate simulation across specialties and disciplines, as well as potentially reduce the workload on specific individuals.
- Closer relationships among decision-makers. A statewide simulation system, by raising awareness of programs throughout a state, helps make decision-makers more knowledgeable and more likely to be sensitive about the consequences of decisions, which may help make economic or resource decisions less contentious.
- Better access to expertise. With a statewide system in place, smaller programs and those at nonacademic centers may be better able to gain access to content experts or administrative advice not otherwise available. A statewide system also fosters a migration of expertise from primarily academic settings to the private and nonacademic sectors. Such migration is important for sustainability.
- More opportunities to train trainers. One of the greatest hurdles to simulation is the shortage of personnel trained in the content of simulations and in the administration of simulations. Simulation sites will not be able to expand without a mechanism for training additional experts to deliver these services. A statewide system can provide diverse opportunities for such training.
- More cost sharing. With a statewide system, some costs can be shared among groups for physical facilities, staffing resources, and content experts. For instance, if a rural location would like to create a simulation site, but only needs the use of a manikin and technical expert a few days a month, a statewide system may make it feasible to contract for those services from another site.
- Increased opportunities for applications. As more trainers and sites come on line in a statewide system, the possible applications of simulation increase (eg, certification).
- Common curriculum. With various sites teaching a common curriculum in a statewide system, education should become more standardized, which in turn should, in combination with shared expertise, improve the quality of education available at any given site.
- Saving time. Developing a curriculum consumes time and resources. Through sharing of curriculum across a network in a statewide system, each site can benefit from not having to "reinvent the wheel."

- Stronger purchasing power. Statewide systems can reduce overall costs by allowing larger-scale purchases with lower per-unit prices, and by reducing the absolute number of purchases as facilities share equipment.
- More power to influence industry. Requests to companies providing simulation equipment for changes in programming or capabilities are much likelier to be heeded from a large system, such as a statewide system, representing multiple end-users.
- Greater anesthesia practice collaboration. States, by recognizing and supporting simulation centers as a part of the educational system, not only increase capacity and quality, but, as the benefits of networking become obvious, help bridge the chasm between academic and nonacademic practices. In contemplating the use of simulation for credentialing, capacity becomes immediately problematic. Were simulation to be required for either board certification or maintenance of certification, the number of individuals needing testing would virtually overwhelm the sites currently functioning at the level required. By facilitating robust growth, statewide networks can help in this arena.
- National significance. Statewide models can be useful nationally. As professions move forward, an inevitable push to standardize curriculum and delivery will emerge. This will become particularly important as maintenance of certification and residency programs start to incorporate simulation. As described in the ASA white paper on simulation, a mechanism for certifying and overseeing simulation sites will quickly become necessary if the sites are to be used for certifying or credentialing providers. The steps taken to develop statewide systems, with inevitable successes and failures in creating consensus and broad applicability, will inform the development of this sort of oversight. A national model, specialty-specific or multidisciplinary, that respects state diversity is possible, but likely at least 10 years away.

Governance and standards

Economies are gained by decreasing redundancy and creating uniformity where uniformity is of benefit. Our medical education systems, graduate and postgraduate, are based to some degree on these principles, and simulation cannot be an exception. Further, confidence that individuals are receiving a high standard of education irrespective of educator lends tremendous credibility to the process.

Though the creation of standards and a common curriculum can be a gargantuan feat, it can be accomplished through structures that encourage and even reward collaboration. This is the key to statewide simulation. The notion that people feel they are part owners of something bigger can be a strong motivator. What seemed gargantuan appears more manageable when many willing parties are involved. Also, the notion of sharing can be intimidating, as all participants naturally try to protect what is theirs. Breaking this barrier by defining success at a state level rather than at an individual level is critical.

No system is perfect. Applying simulation statewide has pitfalls and disadvantages, the most obvious being sheer size. Though there are a myriad of possible approaches to management, the primary distinction to be made is between those with authority to issue requirements (the governing model) and those without (the nongoverning model).

Standards are easier to implement and enforce in a model with central governance. The question, however, is whether such benefits outweigh the costs. First, one cannot presume all potential participants will buy in to the notion of central governance. It is challenging to implement governance without some form of executive mandate, such as a state law. Further, traditional budgets and allocations are not yet set to accommodate participation in such a venture. Finally, the loss of a sense of control and ownership by users (ie, centers) creates some degree of backlash. What has been observed nationally is that centers that lack a sense of ownership of processes and decision-making are more likely to circumvent the central structure and follow their own paths. To succeed, then, a governed system must have, in addition to the common need to survive, executive (ie, decision-making–level) buy-in, agreed-upon funding, and consensus throughout. Perhaps we will see this in the future as regulators weigh into the process.

In a nongoverning structure (as in Oregon), programs own and govern themselves. As with governing models, they stress success of simulation as a whole rather than the ascendancy of any one program. Though they cannot demand participation, individuals come to the table because of the network's power to generate grant money, enable more favorable purchase pricing, facilitate training of trainers, and provide other benefits. A nongoverning model could gain some degree of control if it establishes itself as a must-have entity, and nothing precludes a nongoverning model from morphing to a governing one. However, that would require several other factors to fall into place.

Regardless of the governing structure, some other challenges arise in a statewide system:

- Difficulties with initial costs and forming collaborations. A statewide application can be more cost-effective than multiple separate local initiatives. The northeast region of the United States has many programs. Could money have been saved through greater collaboration? Collaboration is time consuming, and much of the investment is up-front. The benefit of cost savings is only realized later on in the process. It is difficult to ask a hard-working health care provider to put efforts into forming collaborations when the cost benefits will not be gained until far in the future. Developing a system that leverages expertise and resources for a common good will reduce implementation time and, in theory, increase success rates. This has been observed preliminarily in Oregon.

The cost savings in this respect have been significant, although not published. To date $1.3 million has been spent by the Oregon Simulation Alliance to develop simulation programs across the state. This has been focused mainly on transferring expertise to individuals. It is reasonable to assert that individuals with knowledge will be more efficient and cost effective than a novice. This has lead to thoughful institutional investments in their respective programs after there was a clear understanding of the need and process.

- Importance of maintaining local relevance. Properly implemented, a statewide simulation network gives individuals many potential benefits, including those related to program planning, training of trainers, buying power, access to expertise, and actual training opportunities. These issues speak to both capacity and quality. The pool of trained personnel is larger, and those people are more likely to be working from similar standards. This is positive as long as the system is constructed to remain open to fresh and new ideas. Having the capacity to provide simulation education opportunities to most anesthesiologists in the state (often locally) allows programs to provide content that is more locally relevant and, one could argue, more economically palatable. Similarly, a simulation program that is locally housed can help ensure that local practice standards are taught and met. If curricula are not tailored to the practice environment of the physician, concepts being taught may be irrelevant or contrary to the policies of the hospital in which the physician works.

Statewide needs analysis

So why is knowledge of simulation-related market forces important? Our practices, from the most business-oriented to the most academic, are all driven by market forces to some extent. Therefore, knowing why simulation is going to happen helps us prepare and lead the process rather than have the process defined for us.

Similarly, to understand statewide simulation, one needs to understand what forces are moving simulation forward. This market analysis is a basic business principle. Simply presuming those who have simulation expertise know what needs exist in a large-scale endeavor can be both fallacious and costly. In the last decade many have attempted to move simulation forward by showing that simulation affects outcomes. This is an elusive endpoint. Paradoxically, simulation education is seeing exponential growth despite the lack of outcome data. This is not surprising as other industries, such as aviation, have adopted simulation more on psychometric and fiscal data rather than on outcome data.

So what is pushing simulation forward? The health care market is. Our industry is facing several challenges at a fiscal, regulatory, and safety level.

As the cost of health care rises, consumers, insurance companies, and governmental organizations are expecting the best education for physicians to give better patient care with fewer mistakes. Simulation is being viewed as a tool to confront these challenges. Within undergraduate medical education, the United States Medical Licensing Examination started using simulated patients to assess and certify clinical skills beginning with the class of 2005. Graduate medical education's adoption of core competencies into curricular requirements has led to a new awareness of the importance of professionalism, judgment, thinking, and communication skills. Simulation, especially manikin-based, addresses these areas consistently. It provides a venue for practicing these skills, which were otherwise practiced through direct patient contact. Each of these skills and competencies is dependent on experience much more than knowledge. The need for tools to address patient safety, new regulatory requirements, and higher standards all point to simulation. The use of simulation will spawn new research that will help address its impact on outcomes.

It is difficult to foretell the future of simulation. However, one can make some educated predictions. Simulation related to nursing will dominate the field because of the sheer volume of practicing nurses the large number of nurses that need to be trained, and the fact that nurses, have been using a skills lab metaphor for decades. Schools of nursing and hospital-based nursing represent the largest individual segment of the clinical health care workforce. It is not surprising then that hospital-based simulation will be the dominant venue. The hospital setting involves many disciplines and professions, and will therefore also act as a springboard for the use of simulation for graduate medical education and maintenance of certification activities. Schools of medicine will lag, the process of curricular change being slower. Allied health has been using simulation for many years. Such use will continue to increase.

Implementation—the structure

Implementation of a statewide simulation network is no simple feat. It requires an organizing body, an understanding of the market, and most obviously a business plan that is consistent with the need and fiscal reality of the market. A discussion of the Oregon implementation strategy and market assessment outcomes illuminates the complexity of implementation.

Through representation of many entities with common and different needs, the Oregon Simulation Alliance (OSA) was established in 2003 and incorporated as a not-for-profit in 2005 (Fig. 1). The original group morphed into a governing council, in the form of a board of directors, which oversees all the functions of the OSA. The OSA itself does not provide service directly but rather acts to evaluate needs, create access, and develop strategies to address the needs. Services are outsourced and provided by outside entities with specific and relevant expertise. A Web site that acts as an

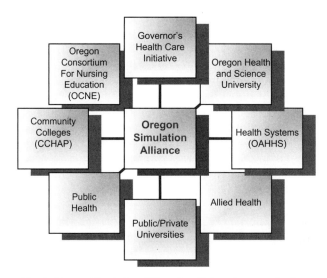

Fig. 1. Oregon Simulation Alliance's collaborative organizations.

information portal (www.oregonsim.org) reflects the OSA's natural evolution. The goal of the alliance is to create a system of access that will result in a large simulation talent pool that will ensure a sustainable future. This also expands the breadth of expertise.

The OSA, as a nongoverning organization, leaves program decisions to local entities. The only time the OSA imposes requirements is when it provides financial assistance to a program. The requirements are not onerous and involve minimum standards and use expectations. In this way programs are not burdened by the traditional morass of reporting requirements of traditional funding sources. Programs are expected to police themselves. This is effective in a state the size of Oregon. The OSA negotiates with vendors for favorable pricing to bring the best value to Oregon programs.

In dealing with organizations with revenue-generating interests, this collaborative approach was initially appealing but later became a threat. Competitive processes always exist and exert pressure on the system. The presence of such organizations is not especially problematic as long as the revenue-generating organizations represent a minority of participating organizations, which they do, and as long as they do not exert undue influence on the collaborative process. Failure to acknowledge them, however, will almost certainly increase risk for any collaborative.

The principles developed in part by the OSA are critical in allowing Oregon anesthesiologists to collaborate in an implementation pertinent to their practices. There are current discussions that would create a collaborative among >75% of the state's practicing anesthesiologists and all of the state's anesthesia residents.

Implementation—site assessments

As alluded to earlier, for any large enterprise to work, its leaders must understand their market and the available infrastructure. Without due diligence, assumptions are made that may prove costly in the long run. The OSA recognized that in-depth assessment of collaboratives and sites interested in simulation would give it access to information that would guide its statewide implementation strategy. The assessment was not a technology review but a comprehensive evaluation of readiness for simulation. The evaluation delved into experience, business planning, infrastructure, and governance. The resultant data were telling (Fig. 2) [8], showing the expected high level of desire and space allocation but a very low level of business planning, true collaboration, funding, and concrete executive directive (not simply soft support).

In the case of simulation use for local or national certification processes, site assessments may also be a part of quality assurance for the educational product delivered. To have significance, the simulation experiences must be recognized as consistent and full of high-quality and meaningful content. In addition, steps must be taken to deliver to legislators and providers of support to simulation centers some "return," including the assurance that the quality is there in the end product. Recently, Oregon state legislators toured simulation facilities to increase their understanding of how the funding was being used. This benefited the legislators by improving their awareness of the potential importance of simulation in medical education and practice. It also benefited the simulation sites by generating continued support.

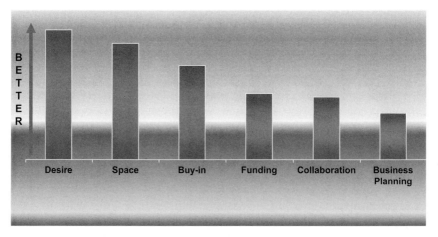

Fig. 2. Results of the Oregon Simulation Alliance's assessment of the level of readiness at sites interested in simulation. (*Courtesy of* SimHealth Consultants, LLC, Portland, OR; with permission.)

Results and consequences—a private and academic partnership example

Optimal implementation for any state depends on local circumstances. Where conditions are favorable, smaller, regional consortiums (ie, covering part of a state) might be nimbler and more responsive to local demands. However, multiple unconnected consortiums in a state may result in wasteful redundancies, added bureaucracies, higher costs, and fewer benefits from economies of scale compared to a comprehensive statewide system. There are now examples of statewide simulation collaboration in obstetrics, schools of nursing, general surgery, and anesthesiology.

In Oregon, the two largest groups of anesthesiologists, the Oregon Anesthesiology Group (190 physicians) and Oregon Health & Science University (60 faculty physicians, 30 residents, 6 fellows), are in discussions to collaborate on implementing simulation opportunities for all members.

The aim is to create an efficient simulation specialist workforce. By employing the classic principle of leveraging existing resources and expertise, the groups will develop a pool of individuals able to deliver quality and diverse simulation education to participants. Cross training of simulation specialists from each group will not only rapidly increase the simulation specialist pool, but will allow individuals from each group to act as external resources for each other for continuing medical education, quality training, and activities related to maintenance of certification.

By cooperating in the design of standards, scenarios, and infrastructure, the resulting collaborative group is also expected to be far more responsive to the diverse needs in a state that is both rural and urban, where groups use both all-physician and care team models, and where many other differences exist. Traditional competitors will have a common purpose in creating a win–win collaboration. It is expected, too, that interdisciplinary opportunities will increase as groups become comfortable with true collaboration.

What will continue to be an issue regardless of the size of the organization superstructure is the need for assurance to the trainee of a quality end-product. Although such certification may come from national certification as discussed earlier, this statewide model is uniquely positioned to accomplish this with greater efficiency and consensus.

Summary

Health care simulation should be considered a top priority. Properly implemented, it can help health care educators address pressing demands in multiple ways:

Patient safety and care will be improved by better preparing students and current practitioners across health professions through predictable and reproducible competency and experience-based learning.

A venue will be provided for skills that can be taught more effectively through practice rather than lecture.

In this venue, professionals from disparate disciplines can break traditional silos and learn to function within a team environment.

In such an environment, it will be safe to practice, make errors, and learn from them without harming patients.

Through more efficient learning, the number of students in health care education programs could significantly increase, alleviating the growing shortages in nursing, allied health, and medical programs.

Oregon has developed a unique collaboration between health care institutions, state bodies, and educational organizations designed to expand the simulation capacity in the state by garnering funding and sharing resources. This is a model that shows promise in Oregon, but may not necessarily be exportable per se to other states.

An effective collaboration can be powerful and realize considerable gains in efficiency and cost. Anesthesiology in Oregon is positioning itself to introduce such a collaboration. This likely could not have happened without the preparatory work of the OSA.

Whether or not a statewide model is the best model for organization and implementation, the basic underlying concepts are valid at virtually any level—institutional, citywide, regional, or national. The benefits of sharing resources, expertise, infrastructure, and personnel are not new to other industries. The specialty should look at these concepts and seek to overcome barriers, real or perceived. As simulation becomes an integral part of training and continuing education at multiple levels, hospitals and education systems will likely require their own facilities to meet capacity needs. Existing collaborative networks will make this transition smoother and more cost-effective.

References

[1] Joint Commission on Accreditation of Healthcare Organizations. Health care at the crossroads: strategies for addressing the evolving nursing crisis. 2002. Available at: http://www.jointcommission.org/Nurses/nurse-staffing.htm. Accessed April 2007.
[2] Kohn KT, Corrigan JM, Donaldson MS, editors. To err is human: building a safer health system. Committee on Quality of Health Care in America, Institute of Medicin. Washington, DC: National Academy Press; 1999.
[3] Jeffries PR. A framework for designing, implementing, and evaluating simulations used as teaching strategies in nursing. Nurs Educ Perspect 2005;26(2):96–103.
[4] Seropian MA, Brown K, Gavilanes JS, et al. An approach to simulation program development. J Nurs Educ 2004;43(4):170–4.
[5] Issenberg SB, McGaghie WC, Petrusa ER, et al. Features and uses of high-fidelity medical simulations that lead to effective learning: a BEME systematic review. Med Teach 2005; 27(1):10–28.
[6] ASA Workgroup on Simulation Education. ASA approval of simulation programs. 2006. Available at: http://www.asahq.org/ASASimWhitePaper031506.pdf. Accessed April 2007.
[7] METI to Deliver State-of-the-Art Technology to New Jersey Department of Health & Senior Services for Statewide Disaster Medicine and Homeland Security Program. Available at: http://www.meti.com/downloads/NJ.pdf. Accessed April 2007.
[8] Seropian MA, Driggers B. The Oregon simulation readiness assessment—evaluating the initial steps of the Oregon simulation implementation model. 2005.

ELSEVIER
SAUNDERS

Anesthesiology Clin
25 (2007) 283–300

ANESTHESIOLOGY
CLINICS

Crew Resource Management and Team Training

Eswar Sundar, MD[a],*, Sugantha Sundar, MD[a],
John Pawlowski, MD, PhD[a], Richard Blum, MD[b],
David Feinstein, MD[a], Stephen Pratt, MD[a]

[a]Department of Anesthesiology, Harvard Medical School, Beth Israel Deaconess Medical
Center, CC-539, 1 Deaconess Road, Boston, MA 02215, USA
[b]Department of Anesthesia, Perioperative and Pain Medicine, Harvard Medical School,
Childrens Hospital, 300 Longwood Avenue, Boston, MA 02115, USA

Health care professionals work in a complex environment. Care of patients in high-acuity areas, such as intensive care units, emergency rooms, operating rooms, and labor and delivery suites, require the constant input of expertise from individuals with varying backgrounds and training. Anesthesiologists, nurses, surgeons, pediatricians, intensivists, respiratory therapists, attendants, and technicians need to work with each other to deliver care in the safest possible manner. Yet, when these highly qualified individuals train in their formative years, hardly any attention is spent on role crossover and they often do not have a clear appreciation of each other's priorities and responsibilities. Health care professionals have long been ingrained to function as responsible individual experts taking responsibility, credit, and blame for individual actions.

High-reliability organizations (HROs) are institutions where individuals, working together in high-acuity situations facing great potential for error and disastrous consequences, consistently deliver care and positive results with minimal errors. Health care today in the United States can hardly qualify as an HRO [1].

Stephen Pratt is a consultant to Team Performance Plus, a division of Risk Management Foundation of the Harvard Medical Institutions Inc. and shareholder of Patient Safety Training Group LLC. Other authors of this paper have no financial interests in the subject of this article.

* Corresponding author.

 E-mail address: esundar@bidmc.harvard.edu (E. Sundar).

doi:10.1016/j.anclin.2007.03.011
anesthesiology.theclinics.com

In 2000, the Institutes of Medicine released a sentinel report, To Err is Human: Building a Safer Health System [2]. The report dealt with the issues of medical errors and patient safety within health care organizations. This report published for the first time the often-repeated statistic that 44,000 to 98,000 patients in American hospitals die each year as a result of avoidable medical errors. The report pointedly stated that "health care is a decade or more behind other high-risk industries in its attention to ensuring basic safety." A frenzy of public debate and media attention on the state of American health care institutions prompted President Bill Clinton to sign an executive order to require federal departments to come up with a list of recommendations to make health care safer [3,4]. The Institutes of Medicine report made a number of recommendations, including the implementation of teamwork-based approaches following the example of the aviation industry [2]. The report specifically recommended that initiatives be undertaken within the health care arena to set up team training programs based on aviation's crew resource management programs. The report also supported the use of simulation-based education and training. Team training has also been advocated by other organizations, such as the Joint Commission on Accreditation for Healthcare Organizations (JCAHO) [4].

Principles of team training

Early forays into team training started in the 1950s and 1960s, predominantly in the military. Most of the drive behind team training resulted from the review of accidents and failures. In the 1990s, the philosophy behind team training was based largely on the concept of a "shared mental model." Mental models are knowledge and mechanisms that can be leveraged to describe, explain, and predict events. Effective teams typically use a shared mental model to achieve a mutually agreed upon goal in the safest possible manner [5]. To work effectively together, team members must also possess appropriate knowledge, skills, and attitudes; such as skills in monitoring each other's performance, knowledge of their own and their teammates' responsibilities, and a positive disposition toward working in a team [1].

Crew resource management is one of the most popular adaptations of the shared mental model of team training. Crew resource management has been used for many years in the aviation industry and has been generally shown to produce positive reactions, enhance learning, and promote desired behavioral changes [6,7]. Crew resource management in aviation is not standardized and different training programs exist for different commercial and military aviation applications. In general, most crew resource management training programs encompass team training sessions, simulation exercises, interactive group debriefings, and measurements of aircrew performance [8,9]. Also, crew resource management programs may teach aviation crews about human limitations and involve participants in assessments of their own behavior and the behavior of peers. Concepts taught include those related to making inquiries, seeking relevant data, advocating actions, communicating proposed action plans, resolving conflicts, and making decisions. Additionally, participants learn to understand cognitive errors and are taught how stressors, such as fatigue, crisis, and work overload, contribute to human error.

Elements of crew resource management include briefings, conflict resolution procedures, and performance reviews.

A briefing is a short summary of the proposed action or procedure. During a briefing, safety issues are discussed and compensatory or corrective action proposed. After a briefing, members of the team are asked to verify their understanding of these plans, thus cultivating the formation of a shared mental model [10,11].

Conflict resolution is employed when the actions of other members of the team are questioned following the perception that safety concerns are not being addressed. Members must share a tacit understanding that such challenges are not acts of insubordination or sabotage. The two-challenge rule is an effective nonconfrontational way of asserting a team member's concern [10,12]. In aviation, the concept of the "two-challenge rule" has been institutionalized. The gist of this rule is that if a pilot puts the aircraft in an unsafe condition, the subordinate must challenge the action twice if necessary. If no answers or if nonsensical answers are provided, the subordinate is empowered to take over the controls [13]. In medicine, when there is a conflict among team members, such conflicts must be resolved with the best interests of the patient in mind.

In a performance review, team members verify and monitor the actions of each other and conduct a debriefing about all actions pivotal to the safety of the patient [10,11].

Salas and colleagues [14] identified what they called the "big five" core components of team effectiveness: (1) team leadership, (2) mutual performance monitoring, (3) backup behavior, (4) adaptability, and (5) team orientation. These components and others with their characteristics are presented in Table 1.

Team training using crisis resource management

Many health care organizations have set up team training programs based on the principles of crew resource management. Despite the unproven record of crew resource management principles in the making of an HRO and effective medical teams, most people believe that crew resource management principles are effective and it seems crew resource management in health care is here to stay [1,11,15,16]. The philosophy of crew resource management has been applied to high-acuity environments, such as operating rooms, intensive care units, emergency rooms, labor and delivery suites, and neonatal intensive care units [11,17]. In such environments, crew resource management is called crisis resource management [11,18]. Different

Table 1
Characteristics of effective teams

Team knowledge, skills and attitude	Characteristics
Team leadership	Has a clear common purpose
	Establishes team member roles that are clear but not overly rigid
	Involves the right people in decisions
	Conducts effective meetings
	Establishes and revise team goals and plans
	Ensures that team members believe the leaders care about them
	Distributes and assign work thoughtfully
Backup behavior	Compensates for each member
	Manages conflict well; makes certain that team members confront each other effectively
	Regularly provides feedback (debriefings) to each member, both individually and as part of a team
	Deals with poor performers
	Incorporates self-correcting techniques
Mutual performance monitoring	Effectively "spans" boundaries to reach stakeholders outside the team
	Ensures that members understand each others' roles and how they fit together
	Examines and adjusts the team's physical workplace
	Periodically diagnoses team effectiveness, including its results
Communication	Communicates often enough
Adaptability	Ensures that members anticipate each other
	Reallocates functions as needed
	Recognizes and adjusts strategies under stress
	Consciously integrates new team members
Shared mental models	Coordinates without the need to communicate overtly
Mutual trust	Trusts other team members' "intentions"
Team orientation	Selects team members who value teamwork
	Strongly believes in the team's collective ability to succeed

Adapted from Salas E, Sims DE, Klien C. Cooperation and teamwork at work. In: Encyclopedia of applied psychology. Volume 1. Spielberger CD, editor. San Diego (CA): San Diego Academic Press; 2004. p. 500; with permission.

crisis resource management programs have developed key concepts based on crew resource management to facilitate education and training. Most of the key concepts from one program to the next are the same or similar. Murray and Foster [19] identify some of the key concepts of crisis resource management as applied to health care (Box 1).

Leader or event manager

The first person to arrive on the scene may establish himself as the leader or event manager. However, if a person who arrives later has more intimate

Box 1. Key concepts of crisis resource management

Roles
    What is a leader?
        Steps back and manages an event
        Sets clear goals
        Organizes the team
        Delegates responsibility
        Distributes work appropriately
    What is a follower?
        Assumes assigned responsibility
        Feeds back event management data
        Provides task and cognitive support
        "Owns" delegated problems
    Roles can be exchanged
    Communication
        Address people directly: introduce yourself
        Declare an emergency: urgency, not panic
        Establish your communication paths
        Use nonjudgmental comments
        Close the loop: give feedback
    Global assessment
        Steps back: physically and mentally
        Steps back to see the whole picture
        Delivers verbal review of patient and situation
            Avoids fixation errors
            Provides clarity of ideas
            Generates new ideas
    Support
        Know that asking for help when needed is a sign of maturity,
            not of weakness
        Understand that incremental help may be called
        Identify sources of help available?
        Know when and whom to call for help
        Ascertain the type of help needed: advice? hands-on?
            specialized?
    Resources
        Prepare for anticipated needs: special carts, memo sheets
        Understand the infrastructure
        Know how support systems work
        Promote internal and external thinking "outside the box"

Modified from Murray WB, Foster PA. Crisis resource management among strangers: principles of organizing a multidisciplinary group for crisis resource management. J Clin Anesth 2000;12(8):634; with permission.

knowledge of the patient, it may be more appropriate for that person to take over the leadership role.

The event manager should stand back and not get involved in physically doing any task. Instead, the event manager should focus on directing individual tasks to team members. The event manager or leader constantly assimilates information from team members and should never lose sight of the "big picture."

Members

Members are not necessarily the junior members on the team. Members are most often the persons most suited for specific tasks. For example, airway management may best be assigned to an anesthesiologist. Chest tube placement may best be assigned to a surgeon. There should be constant open discussions and updates between the leader and the members. Members should be careful not to usurp the role of the event manager but stick to their given task and try to centralize communication through the team leader to maximize team situation awareness as opposed to communicating directly with other members.

Communication

The JCAHO analysis of sentinel events and root causes lists lack of effective communication as the number one reason for the occurrence of sentinel events [20]. Similarly, 70% of commercial flight accidents are attributed to errors of communication among crew members [21]. Effective communication involves addressing people by their given names and making eye contact. Closing the communication loop by repeating orders is vital to ensure that requests have been heard correctly and acknowledged. Feedback from team members to the person in charge allows constant reassessment of the situation. The SBAR tool advocated by Leonard and colleagues [21] is an effective method for ensuring uniformity in communication. SBAR stands for situation, background, assessment, and recommendation. Each of the four words corresponds to a question that must be addressed: Situation—what is going on with the patient? Background— what is the clinical background or context? Assessment—what do I think the problem is? and Recommendation—what would I do to correct it?

Global assessment

Leaders and event managers should constantly step back and take in the "big picture" without getting fixated on individual acts. The team should believe that the actions being taken are in the best interest of the patient and anticipate a positive response if correct management plans are being implemented and followed. When desired results are not forthcoming, it is worthwhile to do a "reality check" and question the assumptions and conditions on which the management plan was based.

Resources and support structures

The team and the leader should constantly assess the resources available to them. Making full use of the support available is critical. For example, an attendant may not be proficient at inserting an intravenous line but can be asked to prepare medications, such as dantrolene in a malignant hyperthermia crisis. The leader should not shy away from requesting fresh resources and ideas. For example, in a situation involving a massive pulmonary embolism, it may be worthwhile to summon a cardiothoracic surgeon who may not be present initially in the room.

Guidelines for establishing medical team training and improving the safety culture of an organization

The development of an HRO does not happen easily. Development of medical teams can enhance safety within organizations and make the organization more reliable. These transformations require vision, change of culture, and leadership. King and colleagues [22] based their team training model on the work of Salas and Cannon-Bowers [23], Kilpatrick, [24] and Kotter [25]. The model was prepared for the Department of Defense and later modified for medical teams. Health care organizations wishing to implement medical team training are referred to these excellent publications. King and colleagues [22] advocate the following steps in developing a model for building a team to drive change in the safety culture and the formation of an HRO.

Establish a vision

The first step is for leaders to create a long-term vision of improving the culture of safety within an organization. Hospital administrators and department heads must show commitment to this goal and must bring leadership to the task of improving patient safety through team training. This vision will become the mental model shared by staff during encounters with patients.

Plan and prepare the environment

Once a vision or a shared mental model is agreed upon, a change team can be assembled. The change team identifies and develops training and implementation strategies, taking into account the organization's strengths, weaknesses, opportunities, and threats. These strategies include establishing team expectations, setting performance goals, conducting training, and implementing correct team behavior. The change team could consider organizational reorganization; changes in leadership, personnel or performance expectations; job restructuring; work redesign; or even layoffs.

Planning requires a site assessment. The goal of a site assessment is to acquire information regarding currently existing or anticipated factors that might influence teamwork at a facility, to provide information used to customize the training and implementation effort, and to establish and incorporate into practice the tools and processes necessary for ongoing impact and evaluation.

Train and implement behaviors and expectations

The actual process of team training often involves a "train the trainer" approach. Home-grown team trainers or an external organization may be involved in training the first generation of teams. The first generation may be leaders in their respective departments or their assignees. Once formed, leaders then proceed to train other caregivers within the organization. Reenactments, role-playing and low- and high-fidelity simulation may all be used as team training strategies.

Monitor and coach to sustain behaviors

Monitoring involves feedback from team members as well as real-time monitoring and evaluation of team behaviors, which is communicated to leaders, the change team, and staff through a systems feedback loop. Evaluation is built into the support process with posttraining teamwork assessment and safety culture assessment.

Align and integrate the behaviors

The final phase of successful team training is to instill the culture of safety and the team-based approach to crisis or situational management as part of the work ethic just as crew resource management is now an indispensable part of an aviator's job.

Types of medical team training programs

Team training programs were traditionally divided into two types [26]. The following are some of the programs found in a literature search and may not be an exhaustive list. These programs provide training to external organizations and personnel and some of them are proprietary.

Simulator-based programs
    Anesthesia Crisis Resource Management Program
    Team Oriented Medical Simulation
    Multidisciplinary Obstetric Simulated Emergency Scenarios
Classroom-based programs
    Medical Team Management
    Geriatric Interdisciplinary Team Training
    Managing Obstetric Risk Efficiently OB (MORE OB)
    MedTeams
    Lifewings
    TeamPerformancePlus

Anesthesia Crisis Resource Management Program

The Anesthesia Crisis Resource Management Program , developed by Gaba and colleagues, is perhaps one of the most well known simulator-based team training programs [17,27–32]. The program emphasizes leadership, teamwork, communication, and resource management. Critical incidents happen within a high-risk environment, such as an operating room, an emergency room, or an intensive care unit. Participants are filmed and the video is subsequently used to debrief the team and participants [33]. At Harvard Medical School, those trained by the Anesthesia Crisis Resource Management Program are given a reduction in malpractice premiums by Harvard's self-insurer, the Risk Management Foundation [34,35]. Participants are mostly anesthesiologists both at the attending-staff and resident levels. Physicians from other specialties, such as emergency medicine, obstetrics, surgery, radiology and internal medicine, have recently also participated separately in this course [36,37].

Team Oriented Medical Simulation

Crew resource management principles were used in Kantonsspital, University of Basel, Switzerland, to develop the Team Oriented Medical Simulation program. Unlike the Anesthesia Crisis Resource Management Program, where participants from different specialties do not intermingle during a simulation, the Team Oriented Medical Simulation program includes a variety of operating room personnel, such as surgeons, nurses, and support personnel, participating in the simulation simultaneously [38]. The simulated operating room contains the usual anesthetic equipment, linked to a computer. In addition, the manikin has a special abdominal segment that allows the surgeon to perform laparoscopic surgery on pig organs. Team Oriented Medical Simulation is designed to be a 3-hour course. The first hour covers key teamwork concepts, such as communication, resource management, and leadership. This session is followed by a combined surgical and anesthetic simulation. The last hour is spent on debriefing using videotapes on the team's performance and offering suggestions for improvement [39].

Multidisciplinary Obstetric Emergency Scenarios

Multidisciplinary Obstetric Emergency Scenarios was developed by the St. Bartholomew Hospital and the London Simulator [40]. Multidisciplinary Obstetric Emergency Scenarios teaches multidisciplinary teamwork and the impact of human behavior on crisis management. Obstetricians, midwives, and anesthetists participate in high-fidelity simulations of obstetrical scenarios. The participants are videotaped and then debriefed at the end of the session by trained experts. According to an initial evaluation, this program appears to be promising [40].

Medical Team Management

Medical Team Management was developed by the United States Air Force to address the issue of medical errors within Air Force health care facilities [39]. Medical Team Management training aims to reduce medical errors by focusing on human factors associated with teamwork [38]. The Medical Team Management course is a 3-day affair using seven modules based on the previously described "train the trainer" philosophy and includes teaching crew resource management concepts and communications issues [26].

Geriatric Interdisciplinary Team Training

Geriatric Interdisciplinary Team Training includes a day course in skills development and self-evaluations. Geriatric Interdisciplinary Team Training makes use of Teams Signature technology to help each team understand its own level of cohesion, leadership, diversity, and other relevant characteristics [26]. The Geriatric Interdisciplinary Team Training curriculum has 10 didactic sessions. The clinical component of Geriatric Interdisciplinary Team Training is offered in a variety of health care settings, including in-patient rehabilitation services, primary care clinics, day care facilities, home health care sites, and hospice centers. At these clinical settings, Geriatric Interdisciplinary Team Training trainees are given opportunities to visit with and assess real patients, advise on problems and needs, and participate in interdisciplinary team meetings. Unlike other programs, Geriatric Interdisciplinary Team Training does not seem to place heavy emphasis on crew resource management principles.

Proprietary team training programs

A number of proprietary team training programs are now available. Most of them base their programs on crew resource management principles and many of them have not been independently evaluated or compared. The following are some programs found during an Internet search and their mention here should not be construed as an endorsement.

MORE OB

MORE OB is a team training program developed by the Society of Obstetricians and Gynecologists of Canada, London, Ontario. The program is directed toward health care personnel involved in the care of the parturient and the newborn. The program has three core modules to be completed by personnel over 3 years and there is an ongoing fourth module building on successes.

MedTeams

MedTeams was developed by Dynamic Research Corporation, Boston, Massachusetts [41]. It was originally created as a program for emergency room medical team management [42,43]. Modifications are now available for operation rooms and labor and delivery suites. After completing the course, primary trainers get certified as MedTeams-certified instructors. MedTeams training consists of seven dimensions important for effective teamwork. About 48 behaviors are identified within these dimensions and measurement tools called Behaviorally Anchored Rating Scales were developed to assess these behaviors [44].

LifeWings

LifeWings, offered by Crew Training International, Memphis, Tennessee, offers programs to enhance patient safety and reduce medical errors, to improve trainee skills in team-building, and to counter the effects of stress. Former aviation pilots lead the training, which includes classroom discussions; role-playing; and guidance on resource management, conflict resolution, and dealing with stress and fatigue. A challenge-and-respond checklist is available for use in the operating room [26].

TeamPerformancePlus

TeamPerformancePlus, Boston, Massachusetts, offers team training in the context of obstetric care [35]. The team has three phases in the implementation of team training based on crew resource management concepts.

Other medical team training programs

Many large health care organizations have developed their own internal medical team training programs. The National Center for Patient Safety was established under the US Department of Veterans Affairs in 1999. The National Center for Patient Safety has been the leader in many patient safety initiatives including medical team training at all Veterans Administration Hospitals [45]. The National Center for Patient Safety team training program is also based on crew resource management principles. The Kaiser Permanente National Patient Safety Program is another example of a program that has put in place a number of safety initiatives, including the management of a preoperative briefing checklist [21,46].

The effectiveness of simulation-based team training

Simulation-based training provides opportunities for trainees to develop requisite competencies through practice in a simulated environment that is representative of actual operational conditions. Trainees also receive feedback related to specific events that occur during training. Successful simulation-based training programs provide opportunities for evaluating team members on multiple levels. History taking, making an inventory of the skills and competencies available within the team, and using them effectively are key areas. Simulation programs must also critically look at individual performances, as well as overall team dynamics, and debrief at the end with appropriate feedback [47].

Byrne and Greaves [48] studied assessment instruments used to measure performance during anesthesia simulation and concluded that the effectiveness of methodologies used for assessing performance during simulation is largely undetermined. A study by Devitt and colleagues [49,50] assessed whether a simulator-based performance evaluation could demonstrate construct validity (the extent to which a test reflects the concepts being learned) and realism. They found that certain scenarios could discriminate skill levels between anesthesia residents and staff without loss of realism. Devitt and colleagues [51] also looked at the issue of fidelity among different raters observing the same simulated anesthesia event on video. They found that there was considerable interrater agreement in the study. Gaba and colleagues [52] concluded in their study that simulation allows for excellent to fair interrater agreement when simulation was used to assess the responses of anesthesiologists to predefined crises. However, one difficulty the raters had was in determining a single score for a participant whose behavior varied over time.

Blum and colleagues [53] used information probes to assess the effectiveness of sharing vital pieces of patient information during a simulated crisis among participants. The average information-sharing episodes, irrespective of the type of simulation, was only around 27%. Despite poor information-sharing among the participants, they rated themselves as improved or somewhat improved at the end of the session. Self-ratings of improvement correlated significantly with measured change in group information probe sharing between the beginning and the end of the course. Simulation-based training coupled with intense briefing was shown to improve communication and cooperation skills, months after the training, compared with a control group without briefing [54].

Despite these studies showing construct validity of simulators, it has been difficult to directly measure human performance and teamwork skills within a simulated environment [55,56]. Studies often need to use tests that do not test the range of concepts taught in the curriculum (lack of content validity). No studies yet show an improvement in patient safety after simulation was used for team training. This may be because no team training program using simulation alone has managed to implement team training for all personnel in a given patient care environment, thus diluting the impact of individual simulator-trained members. Despite the weak evidence of its impact on patient outcome, simulation has been widely adopted [18]. Also, as Gaba has said: "The current system of medical education, training, and maintenance of proficiency has itself never been tested rigorously to determine whether it achieves its stated goals; the high level reviews of the performance of the health care industry suggest that it does not" [57]. Why should simulation be held to a different standard?

The effectiveness of didactic classroom team training

One study on the effectiveness of the MedTeams program in reducing errors in the emergency room reported a statistically significant improvement in behaviors between control and experimental groups. The clinical error rate decreased significantly from 30.9% to 4.4% in the experimental group exposed to the MedTeams principle of formal teamwork training. However, the investigators did not report that the raters were blinded to the group to which the caregivers belong nor were these institutions randomly allocated between the control and experimental group [44]. In another study, a complete restructuring of a general-surgery patient-care team with improved communication among team members was associated with a decreased length of patient stay [58]. Caregivers at the Kaiser Permanente group initiated a preoperative briefing project and demonstrated a decrease in wrong-side and wrong-site surgery [46]. Uhlig and colleagues [59] implemented a collaborative care model involving all members of a cardiac care team. Patients were seen simultaneously by all members of the team at rounds. Their results show a decline in death rates from expected levels after the implementation of collaborative care. However, the investigators stated that other changes were made at the same time the collaborative care model was instituted. It is not clear what those other changes were and how they impacted the final results. The labor and delivery team at the Beth Israel Deaconess Medical Center, Boston, Massachusetts, developed a care model based on team training. The investigators reported a significant 50% decrease in an adverse outcome index after implementation of team training compared with the National Perinatal Information Center's repository of adverse outcome indices in 20 other hospitals [35]. The investigators also reported a 50% reduction in money set aside for malpractice damages. Case studies by the American Institutes of Research evaluating MedTeams, LifeWings, and Medical Team Management conclude that they have many desirable features and share many salient concepts. Posttraining evaluations elicited positive responses from participants [26].

Simulation versus didactic classroom-based team training

Does simulation add anything at all to didactic teamwork training? Pratt and Sachs [60] argue against simulation. The expenditure involved in buying or building a simulator [61], plus the costs of running it, and the resources spent freeing up staff to attend the simulator do not justify any purported advantages. In the same journal, Gaba argues that simulation need not be ruinously expensive and that simulation can be staged in real-life settings [62]. Gaba argues that only simulation can provide the near real-life experience necessary to practice teamwork skills and only simulation offers the initial and ongoing training of experienced personnel dealing with highly complex real-life scenarios [63]. Beaubien and Baker [64] argue that simulation does not necessarily refer to high-fidelity simulation, but there are in fact a number of other options, such as case studies and role plays, that can be equally effective if leveraged fully. A study by Shapiro and colleagues [65] looked at the impact of adding simulation to a didactic teamwork curriculum. Although the experimental group exposed to high-fidelity simulation showed a marginal improvement in BARS, it did not reach statistical significance. To the investigators' credit, this is a rare randomized single crossover prospective, blinded, and controlled study, a difficult one to perform in the field of evaluating teamwork training [18].

Future direction of team training

Although there may never be a randomized controlled blinded study comparing the team training process to other traditional methods of working in high-acuity situations, most experts agree that teaching teamwork has value [18]. This is not to say a scientifically rigorous study evaluating team training is not possible. Indeed, such a study should be an objective worth striving for. Many team training programs draw heavily from crew resource management techniques developed in aviation. While crew resource management has been effective in reducing cockpit error, does crew resource management translate well into healthcare [7]?

There is a need to integrate different applications of simulation across different target populations and purposes. Studies need to be done using simulation to evaluate the fundamental aspects of human performance in health care. Macrosimulation, where a simulation application is developed not for the care team but for the entire health care organization, may be needed to assess the global impact of team training on an organization [57].

Because simulation offers realism and exposes the many shortcomings of human behavior under stress, the way forward may be to combine simulation with classroom training and to combine workers from different specialties during simulation to get them to work together [62].

Currently many team training methods are considered proprietary and, hence, may not be easy to compare. Studies are needed to compare teams trained in different methodologies of team training. To perform these comparisons, health care organizations need to develop core competencies that can be then tested after teams have been trained. Studies will eventually have to be done showing that team training not only induces behavioral change among team members but also actually affects the bottom line by reducing medical errors and making health care safer.

Summary

The Institutes of Medicine report on patient safety conditions inside America's health care organizations has given impetus to a number of initiatives, most notably programs to train medical teams. Crew resource management principles borrowed from aviation have been applied to the development of programs, both simulator-based and nonsimulator-based, to train medical teams with the eventual goal of attaining the status of an HRO. High-acuity environments, such as the operating room, the intensive care unit, the emergency room, and the labor and delivery suite, have constantly changing complex environments where it's crucial that all personnel operate with a shared mental model to maintain patient well being and safely deliver health care. A subset of crew resource management concepts when applied to high-acuity situations in health care may be called crisis resource management. A number of team training programs are offered as examples in this review. Currently, it is difficult to suggest that one type of team training is superior to another and studies are needed in this area. Indeed, most classroom-based team training programs have many overlapping principles and concepts and perhaps the important question to be answered is whether the addition of high-fidelity simulation is necessary.

Although some empirical studies show positive outcome after team training, there is little to suggest that these programs and processes actually improve patient safety and outcome. Studies to prove the positive impact of simulation- or classroom-based team training on patient outcome may be difficult to perform but medical team training based on crew resource management principles is here to stay.

References

[1] Baker DP, Day R, Salas E. Teamwork as an essential component of high-reliability organizations. Health Serv Res 2006;41(4 Pt 2):1576–98.

[2] Kohn L, Corrigan J, Donaldson M. To err is human: building a safer health system. Committee on Quality of Health Care in America. Washington, DC: Institutes of Medicine. National Academy Press; 2000.

[3] Altman DE, Clancy C, Blendon RJ. Improving patient safety—five years after the IOM report. N Engl J Med 2004;351(20):2041–3.

[4] O'Leary D. Patient safety: "instilling hospitals with a culture of continuous improvement." Testimony before the Senate Committee on Governmental Affairs. JCAHO, June 11, 2003.

[5] Paris CR, Salas E, Cannon-Bowers JA. Teamwork in multi-person systems: a review and analysis. Ergonomics 2000;43(8):1052–75.

[6] Salas E, Rhodenizer L, Bowers CA. The design and delivery of crew resource management training: exploiting available resources. Hum Factors 2000;42(3):490–511.

[7] Salas E, Burke CS, Bowers CA, et al. Team training in the skies: does crew resource management (CRM) training work? Hum Factors 2001;43(4):641–74.

[8] Lauber JK. Cockpit resource management training. In: Orlady HW, Foushee HC, editor. NASA Conference Proceedings. Vol: 2455, Ames Research Center. Moffet Field (CA), May 6–8, 1986.

[9] Helmreich RL, Merritt AC, Wilhelm JA. The evolution of crew resource management training in commercial aviation. Int J Aviat Psychol 1999;9(1):19–32.

[10] Musson DM, Helmreich RL. Team training and resource management in health care: current issues and future directions. Harvard Health Policy Review 2004;5(1):25–35.

[11] Burke CS, Salas E, Wilson-Donnelly K, et al. How to turn a team of experts into an expert medical team: guidance from the aviation and military communities. Qual Saf Health Care 2004;13(Suppl 1):i96–104.

[12] Macready N. Two-challenge rule averts errors, improves safety. Or Manager 1999;15(1): 12.

[13] Simon R, Pian-Smith M, Raemer D. Challenging superiors in the Healthcare environment. International Meeting on Medical Simulation 2005.

[14] Salas E, Sims DE, Burke CS. Is there a "Big Five" in teamwork. Small Group Research 2005; 36(5):555–99.

[15] Grogan EL, Stiles RA, France DJ, et al. The impact of aviation-based teamwork training on the attitudes of health-care professionals. J Am Coll Surg 2004;199(6):843–8.

[16] Pizzi L, Goldfarb NI, Nash DB. Crew resource management and its applications in medicine. Making health care safer: a critical analysis of patient safety practices. Evidence Report/Technology Assessment 2001;43:503–10.

[17] Gaba DM, Fish KJ, Howard SK. Crisis management in anesthesiology. Philadelphia: Churchill Livingstone; 1994.

[18] Cooper JB. Are simulation and didactic crisis resource management (CRM) training synergistic? Qual Saf Health Care 2004;13(6):413–4.

[19] Murray WB, Foster PA. Crisis resource management among strangers: principles of organizing a multidisciplinary group for crisis resource management. J Clin Anesth 2000;12(8): 633–8.

[20] Joint Commission. Root cause of sentinel events, all categories: 1995–2004. Available at: http://www.jointcommission.org/NR/rdonlyres/FA465646-5F5F-4543-AC8F-E8AF6571E372/0/root_cause_se.jpg, JCAHO, 2006. Accessed December 31, 2006.

[21] Leonard M, Graham S, Bonacum D. The human factor: the critical importance of effective teamwork and communication in providing safe care. Qual Saf Health Care 2004;13(Suppl 1): i85–90.

[22] King HB, Kohsin B, Salisbury M. Systemwide deployment of medical team training: lessons learned in the Department of Defense. In: Advances in patient safety. vol 3. Rockville (MD): Agency for Healthcare Research and Quality. p. 425–35.

[23] Salas E, Cannon-Bowers JA. The anatomy of team training. In: Tobias SJ, Fletcher JD, editors. Training and retraining: a handbook for business, industry, government, and the military. New York: McMillan; 2000. p. 312–35.

[24] Kirkpatrick DL. Evaluating training programs: the four levels. 2nd edition. San Francisco: Berrett-Koehler Publishers Inc; 1998.

[25] Kotter JP. Leading change. Boston: Harvard Business School Press; 1996.

[26] Baker D, Gustafson S, Beaubain M, et al. Medical team training programs in health care. Advances in patient safety; 4:253–67.

[27] Gaba DM, DeAnda A. A comprehensive anesthesia simulation environment: re-creating the operating room for research and training. Anesthesiology 1988;69(3):387–94.

[28] Howard SK, Gaba DM, Fish KJ, et al. Anesthesia crisis resource management training: teaching anesthesiologists to handle critical incidents. Aviat Space Environ Med 1992; 63(9):763–70.

[29] Gaba DM. Improving anesthesiologists' performance by simulating reality. Anesthesiology 1992;76(4):491–4.

[30] Holzman RS, Cooper JB, Gaba DM, et al. Anesthesia crisis resource management: real-life simulation training in operating room crises. J Clin Anesth 1995;7(8):675–87.

[31] Gaba DM. Anaesthesiology as a model for patient safety in health care. BMJ 2000; 320(7237):785–8.

[32] Flanagan B, Nestel D, Joseph M. Making patient safety the focus: crisis resource management in the undergraduate curriculum. Med Educ 2004;38(1):56–66.

[33] Watterson L, Flanagan B, Donovan B, et al. Anaesthetic simulators: training for the broader health-care profession. Aust N Z J Surg 2000;70(10):735–7.

[34] Blum RH, Raemer DB, Carroll JS, et al. Crisis resource management training for an anaesthesia faculty: a new approach to continuing education. Med Educ 2004;38(1):45–55.
[35] Mann S, Marcus R, Sachs BP. Lessons from the cockpit: how team training can reduce errors on L&D. Contemporary Ob gyn 2006;1–7.
[36] Sica GT, Barron DM, Blum R, et al. Computerized realistic simulation: a teaching module for crisis management in radiology. AJR Am J Roentgenol 1999;172(2):301–4.
[37] Reznek M, Smith-Coggins R, Howard S, et al. Emergency medicine crisis resource management (EMCRM): pilot study of a simulation-based crisis management course for emergency medicine. Acad Emerg Med 2003;10(4):386–9.
[38] Helmreich R, Davies J. Human factors in the operating room: interpersonal determinants of safety, efficiency, and morale. Baillieres Clin Anaesthesiol 1996;10(2):277.
[39] Baker DP, Gustafson S, Beaubien J, et al. Medical teamwork and patient safety: the evidence-based relation. AHRQ Publication No. 05-0053. Rockville (MD): Agency for Healthcare Research and Quality; 2005.
[40] Davis C, Gregg A, Thornley D. Initial feedback on MOSES (Multidisciplinary Obstetric Simulated Emergency Scenarios): a course on team training, human behaviour and "fire drills". Anesthesiology 2002;96(Supp 1).
[41] Morey JC, Simon R, Jay GD, et al. A transition from aviation crew resource management to hospital emergency departments: the MedTeams story. Proceedings of the 12th International Symposium on Aviation Psychology. Columbus (OH); 2003.
[42] Simon R, Salisbury M, Wagner G. MedTeams: teamwork advances emergency department effectiveness and reduces medical errors. Ambul Outreach 2000;21–4.
[43] Small SD, Wuerz RC, Simon R, et al. Demonstration of high-fidelity simulation team training for emergency medicine. Acad Emerg Med 1999;6(4):312–23.
[44] Morey J, Robert S, Gregory D, et al. Error reduction and performance improvement in the emergency department through formal teamwork training: evaluation results of the MedTeams project. Health Serv Res 2002;37(6):1553–81.
[45] Neily J, Dunn E, Mills PD. Medical team training-an overview. Topics in Patient Safety 2004;4(5):1–3.
[46] Defontes J, Surbida S. Preoperative safety briefing project. The Permenante Journal 2004; 8(2):21–7.
[47] Salas E, Wilson KA, Burke CS, et al. Using simulation-based training to improve patient safety: what does it take? Jt Comm J Qual Patient Saf 2005;31(7):363–71.
[48] Byrne AJ, Greaves JD. Assessment instruments used during anaesthetic simulation: review of published studies. Br J Anaesth 2001;86(3):445–50.
[49] Devitt JH, Kurrek MM, Cohen MM, et al. Testing internal consistency and construct validity during evaluation of performance in a patient simulator. Anesth Analg 1998;86(6):1160–4.
[50] Devitt JH, Kurrek MM, Cohen MM, et al. The validity of performance assessments using simulation. Anesthesiology 2001;95(1):36–42.
[51] Devitt JH, Kurrek MM, Cohen MM, et al. Testing the raters: inter-rater reliability of standardized anaesthesia simulator performance. Can J Anaesth 1997;44(9):924–8.
[52] Gaba DM, Howard SK, Flanagan B, et al. Assessment of clinical performance during simulated crises using both technical and behavioral ratings. Anesthesiology 1998;89(1): 8–18.
[53] Blum RH, Raemer DB, Carroll JS, et al. A method for measuring the effectiveness of simulation-based team training for improving communication skills. Anesth Analg 2005;100(5): 1375–80.
[54] St Pierre M, Hofinger G, Buerschaper C, et al. Simulator-based modular human factor training in anesthesiology. Concept and results of the module "Communication and Team Cooperation". Anaesthesist 2004;53(2):144–52.
[55] Wright MC, Taekman JM, Endsley MR. Objective measures of situation awareness in a simulated medical environment. Qual Saf Health Care 2004;13(Suppl 1):i65–71.
[56] Baker D, Salas E. Principles for measuring teamwork skills. Hum Factors; 34(4):469–75.

[57] Gaba DM. The future vision of simulation in health care. Qual Saf Health Care 2004; 13(Suppl 1):i2–10.

[58] Friedman DM, Berger DL. Improving team structure and communication: a key to hospital efficiency. Arch Surg 2004;139(11):1194–8.

[59] Uhlig PN, Brown J, Nanson AK, et al. System innovation concord hospital. Jt Comm J Qual Improv 2002;28(12):666–72.

[60] Pratt SD, Sachs BP. Team training: classroom training vs. high-fidelity simulation. Agency for HealthCare Research and Quality. Available at: http://www.webmm.ahrq.gov/perspectives. aspx.

[61] Kurrek MM, Devitt JH. The cost for construction and operation of a simulation centre. Can J Anaesth 1997;44(11):1191–5.

[62] Gaba DM. What does simulation add to team work training? Agency for HealthCare Research and Quality. Available at: http://www.webmm.ahrq.gov/perspectives.aspx.

[63] Gaba DM. Two examples of how to evaluate the impact of new approaches to teaching. Anesthesiology 2002;96(1):1–2.

[64] Beaubien JM, Baker DP. The use of simulation for training teamwork skills in health care: how low can you go? Qual Saf Health Care 2004;13(Suppl 1):i51–6.

[65] Shapiro MJ, Morey JC, Small SD, et al. Simulation based teamwork training for emergency department staff: does it improve clinical team performance when added to an existing didactic teamwork curriculum? Qual Saf Health Care 2004;13(6):417–21.

ELSEVIER
SAUNDERS

ANESTHESIOLOGY
CLINICS

Anesthesiology Clin
25 (2007) 301–319

Simulation: Translation to Improved Team Performance

Elizabeth A. Hunt, MD, MPH[a,*],
Nicole A. Shilkofski, MD[a],
Theodora A. Stavroudis, MD[b],
Kristen L. Nelson, MD[a]

[a]Johns Hopkins Simulation Center, Department of Anesthesiology and Critical
Care Medicine, Johns Hopkins University School of Medicine, 600 North Wolfe Street,
Blalock 904, Baltimore, MD 21287, USA
[b]Johns Hopkins Simulation Center, Department of Pediatrics, Johns Hopkins University
School of Medicine, 600 North Wolfe Street, Nelson 2-133,
Baltimore, MD 21287, USA

The practice of medicine is becoming increasingly complex. No one individual can expect to care for a patient on their own, and must interact with other disciplines and specialties to optimize care. Traditional medical education has emphasized autonomy and, until recently, issues related to teamwork have not been explicitly included in medical curriculum. In addition, medicine has traditionally been very hierarchical, emphasizing a communication structure that follows a chain of command philosophy. Although this type of communication is effective in some realms, it has been shown to contribute to errors in a variety of disciplines.

Recent medical literature highlights that over two thirds of serious medical errors called "sentinel events" and reported to the Joint Commission on Accreditation of Healthcare Organizations were primarily caused by failures in communication [1]. In their 1999 report that showed that as many as 98,000 patients in the United States die each year because of medical errors, the Institute of Medicine highlighted that health care providers tend to be trained as individuals, yet function almost exclusively as teams, creating a gap between training and reality. The Institute of Medicine suggested the use of simulation exercises focused on improving teamwork as one of the mechanisms to improve patient safety [2].

* Corresponding author.
  E-mail address: ehunt@jhmi.edu (E.A. Hunt).

1932-2275/07/$ - see front matter © 2007 Elsevier Inc. All rights reserved.
doi:10.1016/j.anclin.2007.03.004
anesthesiology.theclinics.com

This article reviews important concepts related to teamwork and discusses examples where simulation either could be or has been used to improve teamwork in medical disciplines to enhance patient safety.

Teamwork

Teamwork is a very complex example of human interactions that has been studied at length by organizational and human factors psychologists. A team represents a group of individuals who must work together to perform a common goal. Ideally, a team represents a type of synergy, in that a well-functioning team should be able to do things more effectively, efficiently, reliably, or safely than an individual or a group of individuals working separately could do had they been alone. A poorly functioning team, however, may be antagonistic and detrimental to productivity.

Beaubien and Baker [3] define teamwork as "those behaviors that facilitate effective team member interaction." A review of the medical literature reveals a number of concepts related to teamwork that have now been applied to medicine. Although the terminology regarding these concepts may vary, there are specific behaviors that are repeatedly mentioned and either have been or may be addressed through simulation and are briefly highlighted here (Box 1).

A recurrent theme in teamwork literature is the need for effective communication. The key is to ensure that team members are not merely working alongside one another in parallel, but are actually interacting in a way that makes "the whole greater than the sum of its' parts." Characteristics that enhance effective communication are paramount. For example, a good leader is capable of giving instruction in a manner that ensures that the instruction is heard, understood, and heeded (or if the follower cannot heed the instruction, they communicate that back to the leader).

A practical example

In a series of 35 simulated pediatric medical emergencies (mock codes) conducted on pediatric in-patient wards, in every mock code there was at least one order given by the leader, and assumed to be completed, that was discovered to be incomplete only during debriefing [9]. For example, in scenarios of septic shock, the residents invariably believed that the simulated patient had received 40 to 60 mL/kg of fluid boluses by the end of the 20-minute scenario. On interviewing the nursing staff during debriefing, however, the resident discovered that the nurse had put the bolus on an intravenous pump to run over an hour per usual protocol, because they had not been given a specific instruction in terms of time for completion of the bolus. The nurse further clarified that they had either not heard the instructions for the subsequent boluses or had planned to administer them

Box 1. Characteristics associated with high-performing teams

Situation Awareness (SA): Team performance is improved when team members continually assess their environment and update each other in a process called "shared cognition," so that they are making decisions based on current information and can have a shared mental model of the current state of affairs and an updated plan of action with contingencies. SA allows team to maintain a big picture view of situation. Effective military and aviation teams have higher SA than low-performing teams [4–6].

Leadership: An effective team leader can both command the team and values input from team members. Flattening the hierarchy improves safety because information can flow in both directions, whereas leaders who maintain an authoritarian type of leadership "reinforce large authority gradients, creating unnecessary risk." A leader should try not to perform procedures unless the procedure is essential and no one else is capable of doing it. Stepping back and keeping a bird's eye view allows the leader to take in and process more information and contributes to situational awareness [5–7].

Followership: The nonleader members of the team are called "followers." Good "followership" is just as important for good team functioning as good leadership. Followers need to know their individual role on the team but also contribute to overall team functionality. They must contribute to situational awareness by verbalizing observations about changes in the environment, ideas about diagnosis, to decrease the leaders' workload if necessary, and finally to help the leader avoid mistakes (eg, "the team leader might focus on an incorrect diagnosis and apply the wrong rule [treatment] owing to a fixation error, or be incapacitated, hence everyone in the team should always be alert"). Finally, followers must not assume that the leader knows everything and should feel obligated to share observations that might impact outcome [5,7].

Closed Loop Communication: Closed looped communication is used to ensure that a message that was sent is heeded and understood, and involves "[1] the sender initiating a message, [2] the receiver receiving the message, interpreting it, and acknowledging its receipt, and [3] the sender following up to insure the intended message was received" [4].

Critical Language and Standardized Practices: "Critical language" refers to the use of a catch phrase that means something to

every member of an organization and requires specific action
(standardized practices). United Airlines developed the CUS
program, for "I'm concerned, I'm uncomfortable, this is unsafe,
or I'm scared," and is adopted within the culture as meaning
"we have a serious problem, stop and listen to me." Another
example of a standardized approach to improve the
effectiveness of communication is SBAR (situation,
background, assessment, recommendation). This is a tool that
gives an outline of how "awareness and education regarding
the fact that nurses, physicians, and other clinicians are taught
to communicate in very different styles" [4,6].
Assertive Communication: Safe patient care may depend on the
ability of a team member to speak up and get the attention of
other team members when they believe something might be
going wrong. This is more likely to happen if a team member
believes speaking up will not be held against them. A recurrent
phrase is that people can still show deference to expertise, but
speak up in a "non-threatening and respectful manner." The
idea is all team members may have valuable input, "regardless
of rank." The "hint and hope" model has been described as
a common and dangerous way of trying indirectly to
communicate with other team members [4–6].
Adaptive Behaviors: Teams whose members are flexible and
perform as needed to optimize team functioning and
demonstrate adaptive behaviors are those that can truly benefit
from the synergy of an effective team. Examples of adaptive
behavior that optimize team functionality include: "(a) team
members ask for help when overloaded, (b) team members
monitor each others performance to notice any performance
decreases (mutual performance monitoring), or (c) team
members take an active role in assisting other team members
who are in need of help (backup behavior). An essential
component to the above actions happening is trust among
team members" [4].
Workload Management: Workload management is dependent on
team members demonstrating adaptive behaviors. This
principal requires (1) proper allocation of tasks to individuals;
(2) avoidance of work overloads in self and in others; (3)
prioritization of tasks during periods of high workload; and (4)
preventing nonessential factors from distracting attention from
adherence to protocols, particularly those relating to critical
tasks [5].

Debriefing: Debriefing is the process of reviewing a simulation or real event after it is complete to optimize any lessons that can be learned. When using simulation as a teaching tool, simulation with no debriefing and feedback does not result in effective learning. In terms of real events, teams that debrief themselves afterward have been shown to be higher performing [8].

when the first was done, but did not want to bother the physician to clarify the situation.

Two techniques that can improve communication are for the leader to give the order followed by a specific team member's name to increase the likelihood that the order will be heard, and to use the technique of closed loop communication [4]. The leader gives the command, the follower repeats the command, allowing the leader to know it was heard and interpreted correctly, and the leader confirms what they have heard. Although it is very important that a good leader ensure that their orders have been heard and interpreted correctly, it is equally important that the other team members practice good "followership." They should participate in the closed loop communication, speak up when they are unable to complete the command to improve the team's situational awareness, and use assertive communication techniques to clarify if they do not agree or are concerned about the order. Flattening the hierarchy so that the followers feel comfortable speaking up to the leader is essential to create an environment where followers can point out that they have not yet completed an order or do not agree with the order (see Box 1).

In the previously mentioned case, the resident as team leader was operating on the assumption that the child had received almost 60 mL/kg of fluid boluses and was in some type of fluid-resistant shock, whereas that child had actually received less than 20 mL/kg. This gap between the leader's mental model of the situation and the truth may have a truly negative impact on the child's care and has been observed in reality by the authors when accepting patients in septic shock transferred from various emergency departments. The incongruence between the physician and nursing reports highlights that the team is not on the same page. By debriefing the team members after a real or simulated crisis, however, this lack of situational awareness and closed loop communication can be highlighted and the team members have an opportunity to learn from this mistake. Furthermore, simulation allows the team members to repeat portions of the exercise and to practice communicating with one another until they are truly functioning as a team, all without harming a patient.

In their simulation group, the authors have used simulation as part of an iterative process that allows them to (1) diagnose deficiencies in knowledge, technical skills, or teamwork; (2) create opportunities to practice the deficiency; and

(3) reassess for improvement. The mock codes on the wards revealed this disconnect between the "two islands" (ie, physician and nursing staff). The authors have subsequently used a number of simulation forums to allow pediatric residents and nurses to practice a variety of skills, including those related to teamwork. For example, residents practice giving clear orders for fluid boluses, including explaining out loud their goals of the fluid resuscitation as dictated by shock guidelines, and the nurses practice communicating that they have heard the order and to update the resident when the order has been completed or if they cannot complete the order as directed. Also, an opportunity is taken to explain how fluid can be delivered much faster by pushing with a syringe or using a pressure bag than through a pump, addressing a knowledge deficiency that they can then practice in the next simulation. The key to making these sessions productive is to follow educational principles that highlight the need for having clear educational objectives before each exercise and debriefing afterward to highlight lessons learned and yet to be learned. In this case the objectives might be as follows: (1) knowledge: fluid can be delivered faster by pushing the fluid; (2) technical: actually hook up the IV to a stopcock and IV bag and practice delivering quickly; and (3) teamwork: practice closed loop communication, assertive communication, and situational awareness.

These are just a few of the teamwork characteristics used by highly functioning teams and highlighted in Box 1 and more extensively in the teamwork literature. Now reviewed is the concept of simulation; a brief history, including how aviation transitioned from using simulation for technical skills to prioritizing team training; and examples of teams that can or have used simulation to improve the practice of medicine.

Simulation

Simulation refers to the recreation of an actual event that has previously occurred or could potentially occur. One of the greatest values of simulation is that it can be used over and over again to perfect an action, a procedure, or a conversation without ever exposing the providers or patients to harm. Today, simulation is used in many industries to promote and improve team communication and construction, procedural skill training, educational evaluations, and technologic innovations, such as the usability of devices.

Historical perspective

Leading the way: simulation in aviation

Historically, one of the earliest applications of simulation began with the development of the world's first flight simulator in 1911 by Orville Wright and later with the Link trainer [10,11]. Rolfe and Staples [11] describe the development of flight simulation as a "logical approach to teaching," by using an environment similar to the actual cockpit while still being "safely linked to the ground." Simulation was then used to train pilots how to fly for both military and commercial aviation. Unfortunately, despite technologic advances in aviation and early use of simulation, plane accidents with great loss of human life occurred. To determine why such accidents occurred, it eventually became extremely important to understand the team dynamics in the cockpit. Simulation, however, had not yet been used to evaluate flight team performance or communication; it had only been used to train pilots to fly. When the source of most flight error was eventually determined, the multidimensional aspects of simulation developed.

Transition from technical training to teamwork training

Originally, individual pilot error was most often quoted as the source of aviation-related accidents. In 1979, however, the Aerospace Human Factors Research Division of the National Aeronautics and Space Administration revealed that communication errors, inefficient leadership and coordination skills, and faulty decision-making in crisis situations were more often to blame [12,13]. Accidents were found to be associated with inadequate team communication as opposed to improper individual performance, and shortly thereafter Cockpit Resource Management (CRM) was created [12,13].

Cockpit-crew resource management

CRM is now a well-known, structured curriculum in the aviation industry. The original curriculum was designed to teach flight crews how to communicate effectively as a team and to evaluate their leadership and resource management skills in crisis situations. The focus was the multiperson crew in the cockpit [5]. Subsequent evaluation revealed, however, that critical interactions occurred between the cockpit crew and the remainder of the flight crew, and the name of the program was changed from "Cockpit" to "Crew Resource Management" and is now being applied to all divisions within the aviation industry [5,13].

CRM teaches that all members of a team are vital. If a team member at any level believes that something is not being done appropriately or in the best interest of the team or other people that have put their trust in the team, then that member must speak up. The fact that humans make mistakes, but are able to learn from these errors and prevent their repetition, is an important tenant of CRM training.

CRM uses simulation and team debriefings not only to teach team communication, but also to highlight errors in the simulated setting in the hopes of avoiding the same errors in an actual event involving humans. The cognitive stress associated with crisis situations can be created or recreated through the use of simulated events potentially to determine where, when, and why errors occur in such situations. Over time, commercial pilots were involved in simulations for both the technical and teamwork components of flying, but were only tested on their technical skills, detracting from the importance of the crew training. In the late 1980s, it was recognized that human factors were still contributing to 70% of accidents, and at that time the Advanced Qualification Program, which combined training and testing of both technical and teamwork skills, was implemented [5]. This move represented a huge shift in the approach to training and maintenance of certification for aviation crew members. Teamwork training had become equally important to technical training.

Simulation: application to medicine

Although flight simulation in aviation had its beginnings in 1910, the history of medical simulation using mannequins as partial task trainers dates back to the 1960s with the creation of Resusci-Anne and the Harvey cardiology simulator [14]. Progressively sophisticated and economical computer-driven mannequins, capable of several physiologic actions, have created a more realistic representation of the human patient and are being used for increasing fidelity of simulations used in medical trainings.

The medical community is now highlighting simulation training as the cornerstone to achieving some degree of competence before performing skills on patients, to protect patient safety. The authors' group has coined the phrase "practice on plastic first" to highlight this premise. Although practice is used in this phrase, it is the deliberate practice of a skill in context that is of importance. To achieve perfection of a skill requires dedicated, repetitive training with debriefing to highlight errors or progress.

Simulation for medical team training

David Gaba and others have pioneered the application of simulation training to the medical community, following many of the tenants of aviation training. Gaba and colleagues designed a mannequin-based simulator program known as "Comprehensive Anesthesia Simulation Environment" in the late 1980s. In these situations, human performance was evaluated during anesthesia crisis situations. Application of such evaluations to an anesthesia curriculum resulted in the development of what is now often referred to as "anesthesia crisis resource management" [15,16]. Although originally used in anesthesia, anesthesia crisis resource management has several applications to other divisions within health care, and reference to CRM for the remainder of this article refers to crisis resource management.

CRM training in medicine involves many of the same principles that are found in aviation training, including the three crucial tenants of CRM training: (1) knowledge, (2) practice, and (3) recurrence [17]. Simulated scenarios are used to evaluate team performance in many areas, such as the operating room, trauma bay, and in ICUs, and in events in which small management errors can have grave consequences, such as in cardiopulmonary arrest or in the transport of critically ill patients. CRM training also involves the use of feedback or debriefing sessions as a vital component for process improvement.

The Agency for Healthcare Research and Quality has defined three categories of competencies that are necessary for a team to operate effectively: (1) teamwork-related knowledge, (2) skills, and (3) attitude. Knowledge constitutes an understanding of the requisite skills required for tasks that the team is responsible for, whereas teamwork skills refer to the ability to interact as a team in a proficient and efficient manner. Although these skills are key components of a team, an attitude of trust among members and a desire for improving patient safety are also fundamental to maintenance of a high-quality team [17]. Through the use of simulation, these requisite team components can be rehearsed, allowing team members not only to practice the necessary technical skills, but also to learn to build team trust.

Debriefing

The importance of debriefing after a team simulation experience cannot be overemphasized and is fully reviewed by Randolph elsewhere in this issue. Debriefing allows the team to learn where errors occurred and how they could potentially have been prevented, but it also allows recognition of areas of appropriate performance. Simulation without debriefing has been shown to be ineffective, because errors can be repeated if team members have not been informed that they were making mistakes [8]. In a study by Savoldelli and colleagues [18], those residents who received audio or visual feedback following a simulated scenario performed significantly better on subsequent scenarios than their counterparts who had not received debriefing. Through the use of CRM simulation training and debriefing, health care providers at all levels can learn effective team training in a variety of simulated scenarios, thereby fostering an environment ultimately conducive to patient safety.

Operating room teams

Surgical procedures involve complex, interdisciplinary team communication and have been shown to be responsible for significant morbidity and mortality for patients when errors occur. The operating room can be a highly stressful environment with team members from different disciplines, such as surgery, anesthesia, and nursing, all with different levels of training (attendings, residents, new nurses), who may have met infrequently or never before. Simulation training and debriefing can help the team prepare and anticipate potential adverse events in a complex environment, hopefully avoiding error or subsequently preventing error in repeat interactions.

Simulation in the form of role-playing has been used to practice "time outs" before surgery, to decrease the incidence of wrong site surgery. Actors playing the part of an authoritarian surgeon have been used to train anesthesia and nursing staff how to use assertive communication to enhance patient safety. Simulation has been used to plan complex surgeries, such as separating conjoined twins. At the Johns Hopkins Children's Center, the anesthesia, neurosurgical, plastic surgery, and operating room staff teams worked together to plan a complex surgery including simulating how they would flip the joined children supine in the event of a cardiac arrest while prone. These simulations allowed them to work out problems ahead of time and make sure that they had all the appropriate equipment and job assignments. Varying levels of mannequin-based simulation have also been successfully applied to the operating room arena. Performance assessment of both technical and team communication skills have revealed improved learning through simulation [19,20].

Use of the operating room debriefing tool developed by Makary and colleagues [21] during operating room simulations, as is done after real procedures, may highlight both errors and accolades of an operating room team to determine ways to improve patient safety and give teams practice in using the tool. This tool involves a checklist, to be completed by the team at the completion of a procedure, that allows the team to "assess the cause(s) of an adverse event, near miss or inefficiency." All members of the team are present for this debriefing and are expected to verbalize any concerns pertaining to the case. Implementation of this tool has led to important patient safety modifications. Furthermore, because of its' success in this environment, it is now being applied in other environments outside of the operating room, such as in ICUs.

Obstetric teams

Obstetric teams can also benefit from simulation team training. Difficult deliveries and medical emergencies, such as shoulder dystocia, placental abruption, eclampsia, fetal distress, and multiple gestations, can be simulated with the potential complications associated with each type of event. Through simulation, a labor and delivery room can be recreated and all of the team members can practice their roles, including the obstetrician, anesthesiologist, nurses, and the pediatricians. Thompson and colleagues [22] reported the use of eclampsia drills to identify deficiencies in team preparation for this type of emergency. This type of drill is most effective if all parties that participate in a real event also participate in the simulated events.

Intensive care unit teams

ICUs in adult, pediatric, and neonatal settings are composed of highly dynamic teams that must act quickly in the face of often unanticipated crisis situations. Critically ill patients often require constant physiologic monitoring with complex and evolving technologies. All members of these teams must be trained to manage and communicate effectively and efficiently with these patients and their families. In these circumstances, simulation can provide a replication of the ICU environment, equipped with the technology, including the actual models of equipment that will be encountered in the ICU. Complex scenarios that require successful team interactions can be simulated to help prepare staff for real events, such as cardiopulmonary arrest, difficult airway crises, elevated intracranial pressure, shock scenarios, and the need to "crash onto extracorporeal membrane oxygenation."

Procedures performed in the ICU can also be simulated, such as central venous line insertion, including the gowning procedures to ensure sterility, the technical skill of the insertion itself, and any potential team dynamics. For example, one could create a simulation where a new fellow (actor) is putting in a central line but allows the wire to touch a nonsterile part of the field. The goal of the simulation is for the nurse to notice this break in sterility and use assertive communication tactfully to insist that the fellow stop the procedure until a new wire is available. Another example is to have an ICU physician examine a simulated patient on isolation. The nurse should point out tactfully if the doctor did not wash their hands or put on isolation garb, allowing the team to practice the dynamic of assertive communication that is respectful, but prioritizes the patient's safety over the health care provider's ego. The exercise is repeated until the nurse feels comfortable making the intervention and the physician receives the information with grace and complies with protocols. Team training must focus on both sides of a communication.

Another teamwork issue, lack of leadership, has been sighted as a common error in simulated ICU crisis situations [23]. Lack of leadership often leads to communication mishaps and delays in therapy. The use of didactic education, simulation, and debriefing sessions to replicate such situations have been implemented as part of CRM training at Stanford University for internal medicine trainees rotating through the ICU and have been favorably received as a valuable teaching tool with considerable realism [23].

Another role for simulation in the ICU is to improve communication skills related to discussions about the futility of medical therapy; end-of-life decisions; and the chronicity of medical care, such as long-term mechanical ventilator management and insertion of gastrostomy tubes. Williams [24] ran multidisciplinary ICU teams through simulations with standardized actors playing family members of a person with a severe traumatic brain injury that evolves to brain death. The simulation involved functioning as a team to prepare the family for progression to brain death and then approaching them about organ donation. This exercise was well received by participants and the intervention was associated with increased organ donation rates, presumably because of more effective communication postintervention [24].

Additionally, because ICUs have significant technology that is ever-changing, new devices are often introduced that require retraining of all involved staff. The usability of such complex medical devices can be tested before purchase. In addition, actual models of equipment used in the ICU should be used during team training to increase fidelity. For example, in simulated cardiopulmonary arrests, the authors' team has discovered a lack of familiarity with the defibrillator, particularly the pacing module. They have used simulations of pediatric patients with extremely poor perfusion caused by bradycardia to teach ICU teams how to set up the transcutaneous pacemaker. They purposely do not allow the pacemaker to capture until they have reached a predetermined energy output. They then allow the high-fidelity mannequin to have a slightly improved but not adequate blood pressure. Only if the team notices this and decides to increase the paced heart rate, (because the teams invariably pick a rate that is inadequate for a stressed child) does the child's perfusion improve. This ability to test the interface between medical equipment and personnel during team training is invaluable [25].

Neonatal intensive care unit teams

Studies have identified shortcomings in providers' adherence to the Neonatal Resuscitation Program guidelines [26,27]. In 2000, Carbine and colleagues [26] videotaped neonatal resuscitation skills in the delivery room and found that 54% of 100 neonatal resuscitations deviated from Neonatal Resuscitation Program guidelines. Thomas and colleagues [28] conducted focus groups of nurses, staff nurses, residents, fellows, and attending physicians from the neonatal ICU and found that consistent descriptions of teams or teamwork did not exist. It was noted that hierarchy within groups had a powerful and complicated influence on the way providers communicated with each other, including difficulty in questioning those with authority.

Thomas and colleagues [28] developed 10 behavioral markers for evaluating teamwork in neonatal resuscitation based on standards used in the aviation industry:

1. Information sharing
2. Inquiry
3. Assertion
4. Intentions shared
5. Teaching
6. Evaluation of plans
7. Workload management
8. Vigilance and environmental awareness
9. Overall teamwork
10. Leadership

Using this behavioral marker tool to assess delivery room resuscitations, leadership and assertion were observed in 20% of cases, evaluation of plans in 13% of cases, and intentions stated in only 9% of cases [29]. Moreover, on reviewing 300 videotaped high-risk deliveries at their institution, Finer and Rich [30] also found problems involving teamwork including inappropriate leader and team member activities, inappropriate preparation, communication, and coordination. They suggested that neonatal resuscitation could be improved by the provision of teaching about team and leader functions and encouraged debriefing following complicated resuscitation. Although these studies reveal that certain components of teamwork are lacking in neonatal resuscitations and that this is an area for improvement, further work is needed to decipher the magnitude of this problem and its' effects on delivery room outcomes.

The first high-fidelity simulation-based training program in neonatal resuscitation was developed at Stanford University in the mid-1990s and was well-received by trainees [31]. In addition to emphasizing technical skills, this program also stresses behavioral skills and teamwork skills. Halamek and colleagues showed that trainees believe that this type of training better develops behavioral and critical thinking skills in addition to their technical skills [32]. Currently, a prospective, controlled trial is underway to evaluate objectively the transfer of skills from the simulator to the real environment [32]. Team training courses have also been developed by Ostergaard and colleagues [7] at the Danish Institute for Medical Simulation in response to safety initiatives aimed at improving lack of decision-making skills and absence of teamwork.

Rapid response teams and code teams

A code team or a rapid response team may include people from many disciplines, including physicians (potentially from various specialties); nurses; respiratory therapists; pharmacists; and chaplains. Simulation has been used as both a training tool and as a diagnostic tool to assess how well code or rapid response teams function in their own environment. Evidence gathered from simulated medical emergencies, including cardiopulmonary arrests, demonstrated that these teams were not able efficiently to deliver care; follow appropriate algorithms per American Heart Association Guidelines; or use resuscitation equipment, such as defibrillators, successfully [9,33,34]. These findings were subsequently confirmed in a study of real in-hospital cardiopulmonary arrests [35]. DeVita and colleagues [36] demonstrated that rapid response team training using simulation could improve the functioning of a team and adherence to American Heart Association guidelines.

Transport teams

Both interhospital and intrahospital transport of patients is often necessary. Adequate preparation of such teams is paramount for ensuring patient safety. Studies have shown, however, that teams unfamiliar with the required equipment and the potential adversities that may arise during the transport of patients, particularly those who are critically ill, may lead to an increase in serious complications for the patient [37].

Through the use of simulation, such transport events can be simulated to ensure proper preparation and team communication. Having a team run through a simulated scenario of transporting a patient to the radiology department for a CT scan may reveal previously unrecognized needs. "Is the oxygen tank full, is there a mask of appropriate size available for the intubated patient should the endotracheal tube become dislodged," are common needs on a transport of a critically patient, but can be easily overlooked. The necessary equipment for each transport also needs to be anticipated. Repeated practice can make the tasks more manageable and it is hoped increase the safety of the patient. Furthermore, transport team simulations allow each member to evaluate their roles during the process. Who is going to be responsible for maintaining the IV pumps or who is going to ensure that the end tidal CO_2 monitor is working before and during transport are common tasks that must be assigned and receive follow-up.

Such teams must be able to communicate with one another to ensure that all patient safety features are in place. A transport checklist may assist in ensuring that all jobs have been assigned. The transport team leader should be identified and be ultimately responsible for ensuring the checklist is complete before transport. Both the creation and completion of the checklist can be simulated repeatedly until perfection is achieved. The importance of such collaboration of team members has been highlighted by Flabouris and colleagues [38], who found that good teamwork skills (42%) and good interpersonal communication (4%) were associated with decreased adverse events during transport of critically ill patients. Furthermore, in their review of components of effective neonatal emergency transport networks, Lupton and Pendray [39] cite the importance of establishing team leadership, distribution of workload, stress management, and effective communication among the constituents of a neonatal transport team.

Trauma teams

A trauma team is a cross-functional and multidisciplinary team that can potentially include surgeons, anesthesiologists, intensivists, nurses, respiratory therapists, technicians, and resident physicians. Team membership and function is fluid, depending on patient needs. Trauma teams accomplish their task under a severe information shortage, with patients often brought in unconscious and with little information accompanying them [40]. Simulation can assess both technical performance and behavioral attributes of a team [41].

Several types of simulation have been involved in training trauma teams. The Advanced Trauma Life Support course has variably used animals, partial task trainers, standardized patients, and moulage and high-fidelity mannequin simulators [42]. In addition to skills training, simulation can provide the foundation for team training, including planning, anticipation, establishment of leadership, delegation and distribution of job tasks, consideration of treatment options, review of data, and decision making [42]. Although many simulation studies focus on individual performance, it is widely recognized that optimal trauma care is delivered by experienced and coordinated multidisciplinary teams.

Shapiro and colleagues [43] showed that simulation-based teamwork training improves clinical team performance in an emergency department trauma setting. Their intervention consisted of an 8-hour intensive experience with an emergency department simulator in which scenarios of graduated difficulty were encountered. The experimental team showed a trend toward improvement in the quality of team behavior. In addition, members of the experimental team rated simulation-based training as a useful educational method for enhancing didactic teamwork training. This approach, they concluded, was more representative of clinical care and the proper paradigm in which to perform teamwork training.

Lee and colleagues [44] conducted a study during surgical intern orientation at two academic trauma centers in which interns attended a basic trauma course and were then randomized to trauma assessment practice sessions with either a patient simulator or a moulage patient. Mean trauma assessment scores for simulator-trained intern teams were higher than for moulage-trained intern teams. Marshall and colleagues [45] studied teams of interns who participated in trauma scenarios on a human patient simulator pre and post an Advanced Trauma Life Support provider course and concluded that use of simulation in conjunction with Advanced Trauma Life Support seems to enhance the development of trauma team management skills.

Another study of team behavior in trauma team performance was performed by Holcomb and colleagues [46] using human patient simulators. The study evaluated teams of three members: physicians, nurses, and medics rotating through a civilian trauma center at the beginning and end of the rotation. The 10 teams were compared with expert teams composed of experienced trauma surgeons and nurses. The results showed significant improvement after participation in the rotation, primarily reflecting improved efficiency and coordination of team efforts. The scores of the experimental teams after the rotation approached those of the expert teams. The study concluded that simulation may better prepare teams for the clinical arena, and refresh skills and decision-making processes for uncommon or infrequent occurrences. It also indicates that it is possible to quantify improved performance and to differentiate between experienced and novice teams.

Finally, simulation has been used in emergency departments to diagnose deficiencies in team management of pediatric trauma [47]. A study of simulated mock traumas performed at 35 North Carolina emergency departments revealed problems with pediatric-specific tasks, such as appropriate use of intraosseous needles, weight-based dextrose and volume replacement, and poor preparation for transport to CT. In this study, teams were evaluated to identify possible targets for educational and system-wide interventions that might have the potential to improve the outcomes of pediatric trauma victims [47].

Future directions

The principles of CRM from aviation have been successfully transferred to medical teams. The literature supporting the effectiveness of simulation training to improve teamwork is in the early stages, however, and has not yet been linked to improved patient outcomes. The simulation community must now make a focused effort to use scientific principles to optimize the effect of medical simulation on patient safety. Future use and study of simulation to improve team training should include (1) known educational principles, such as designing curriculum with specific technical and teamwork objectives and use of debriefing; (2) use of existing and development of new validated measures of teamwork as outcome measures; (3) study of decay in teamwork skills so that appropriate intervals for retraining can be determined; and (4) the development of multicenter networks that have the power to detect if team training has an impact on clinical outcomes and patient safety.

Summary

Medical teams require practiced interactions and communications to be effective and efficient. A flattened hierarchy allows for the flow of information to and from the leader. There are a number of teamwork principles that can be practiced to optimize the synergy of a team, including leadership, followership, situational awareness, closed loop communication, critical language and standardized responses, assertive communication, adaptive behaviors, workload management, and debriefing.

The multiple modalities of simulation can be used to optimize team functioning and to ensure achievement of the common goals of these teams, of which patient safety is paramount. "Teams make fewer mistakes than do individuals, and this is especially true when every member of a team is as aware of their teammates' responsibilities as they are their own" [17].

References

[1] Joint Commission on Accreditation of Healthcare Organizations. Joint Commission International Center for Patient Safety. Communication: a critical component in delivering quality care. Available at: http://www.jcrinc.com/publications.asp?durki=10719&;site=153&return=11558. Accessed October 15, 2006.
[2] Kohn LT, Corrigan JM, Donaldson MS. To err is human: building a safer health system. Washington, DC: National Academy Press; 1999.

[3] Beaubien JM, Baker DP. The use of simulation for training teamwork skills in health care: how low can you go? Qual Saf Health Care 2004;13(Suppl 1):i51–6.

[4] Burke CS, Salas E, Wilson-Donnelly K, et al. How to turn a team of experts into an expert medical team: guidance from the aviation and military communities. Qual Saf Health Care 2004;13(Suppl):i96–104.

[5] Hamman WR. The complexity of team training: what we have learned from aviation and its applications to medicine. Qual Saf Health Care 2004;13(Suppl 1):72–9.

[6] Leonard M, Graham S, Bonacum D. The human factor: the critical importance of effective teamwork and communication in providing safe care. Qual Saf Health Care 2004;13(Suppl 1):i85–90.

[7] Ostergaard HT, Ostergaard D, Lippert A. Implementation of team training in medical education in Denmark. Qual Saf Health Care 2004;13(Suppl 1):i91–5.

[8] Issenberg SB, McGaghie WC, Petrusa ER, et al. Features and uses of high-fidelity medical simulations that lead to effective learning: a BEME systematic review. Med Teach 2005;27(1):10–28.

[9] Hunt EA. Simulation of pediatric cardiopulmonary arrests: a report of mock codes performed over a 40 month period focused on assessing delays in important resuscitation maneuvers and types of errors. Presented at the 4th International Meeting on Medical Simulation. Albuquerque (New Mexico), January 2004. Available at: http://www.anestech.org/Publications/IMMS_2004/Hunt.pdf. Accessed October 17, 2006.

[10] Mohler SR. Human factors of powered flight: the Wright brothers' contributions. Aviat Space Environ Med 2004;75(2):184–8.

[11] Rolfe JM, Staples KJ, editors. Flight simulation. Cambridge (England): Cambridge University Press; 1986. p. 14.

[12] Oriol MD. Crew resource management: applications in healthcare organizations. J Nurs Adm 2006;36(9):402–6.

[13] Helmreich RL, Merritt AC, Wilhelm JA. The evolution of Crew Resource Management in training in commercial aviation. Int J Aviat Psychol 1999;9(1):19–32.

[14] Gaba DM. The future vision of simulation in health care. Qual Saf Health Care 2004;13(Suppl 1):i2–10.

[15] Howard SK, Gaba DM, Fish KJ, et al. Anesthesia crisis resource management training: teaching anesthesiologists to handle critical incidents. Aviat Space Environ Med 1992;63(9):763–70.

[16] Cooper JB. Are simulation and didactic crisis resource management (CRM) training synergistic? Qual Saf Health Care 2004;13(6):413–4.

[17] Baker DP, Gustafson S, Beaubien J, et al. Medical teamwork and patient safety: the evidence-based relation. Literature review. Rockville (MD): Agency for Healthcare Research and Quality; April 2005. AHRQ, Publication No. 05-0053. Available at: http://www.ahrq.gov/qual/medteam/. Accessed October 13, 2006.

[18] Savoldelli GL, Naik VN, Park J, et al. Value of debriefing during simulated crisis management: oral versus video-assisted oral feedback. Anesthesiology 2006;105(2):279–85.

[19] Moorthy K, Munz Y, Adams S, et al. A human factors analysis of technical and team skills among surgical trainees during procedural simulations in a simulated operating theatre. Ann Surg 2005;242(5):631–9.

[20] Aggarwal R, Undre S, Moorthy K, et al. The simulated operating theatre: comprehensive training for surgical teams. Qual Saf Health Care 2004;13(Suppl 1):27–32.

[21] Makary MA, Holzmueller CG, Sexton JB, et al. Operating room debriefings. Jt Comm J Qual Patient Saf 2006;32(7):407–10.

[22] Thompson S, Neal S, Clark V. Clinical risk management in obstetrics: eclampsia drills. BMJ 2004;328(7434):269–71.

[23] Lighthall GK, Barr J, Howard SK, et al. Use of a fully simulated intensive care unit environment for critical event management training for internal medicine residents. Crit Care Med 2003;31(10):2437–43.

[24] Williams M. Interdisciplinary experiential training for end-of-life care and organ donation. Presented at the National Consent Conference on Organ Donation. Orlando (FL). April 28–30, 2003.

[25] Hunt EA, Nelson KL, Shilkofski NA. Simulation in medicine: addressing patient safety and improving the interface between healthcare providers and medical technology. Biomed Instrum Technol 2006;40(5):399–404.

[26] Carbine DN, Finer NN, Knodel E, et al. Video recording as a means of evaluating neonatal resuscitation performance. Pediatrics 2000;106(4):654–8.

[27] Thomas EJ, Sexton JB, Lasky RE, et al. Teamwork and quality during neonatal care in the delivery room. J Perinatol 2006;26(3):163–9.

[28] Thomas EJ, Sherwood GD, Mulhollem JL, et al. Working together in the neonatal intensive care unit: provider perspectives. J Perinatol 2004;24(9):552–9.

[29] Thomas EJ, Sexton JB, Helmreich RL. Translating teamwork behaviours from aviation to healthcare: development of behavioural markers for neonatal resuscitation. Qual Saf Health Care 2004;13(Suppl 1):57–64.

[30] Finer NN, Rich W. Neonatal resuscitation: toward improved performance. Resuscitation 2002;53(1):47–51.

[31] Halamek LP, Kaegi DM, Gaba DM, et al. Time for a new paradigm in pediatric medical education: teaching neonatal resuscitation in a simulated delivery room environment. Pediatrics 2000;106(4):E45.

[32] Agency for Healthcare Research and Quality. Disseminating research results: transfer of a novel pediatric simulation program, project number HS12011–01. Available at: http://www.ahrq.gov/qual/newgrants/dissem.htm. Accessed October 17, 2006.

[33] Sullivan MJ, Guyatt GH. Simulated cardiac arrests for monitoring quality of in-hospital resuscitation. Lancet 1986;2(8507):618–20.

[34] Iirola T, Lund VE, Katila AJ, et al. Teaching hospital physicians' skills and knowledge of resuscitation algorithms are deficient. Acta Anaesthesiol Scand 2002;46(9):1150–4.

[35] Abella BS, Alvarado JP, Myklebust H, et al. Quality of cardiopulmonary resuscitation during in-hospital cardiac arrest. JAMA 2005;293(3):305–10.

[36] DeVita MA, Schaefer J, Lutz J, et al. Improving medical emergency team (MET) performance using a novel curriculum and a computerized human patient simulator. Qual Saf Health Care 2005;14(5):326–31.

[37] Vos GD, Nissen AC, Nieman FH, et al. Comparison of interhospital pediatric intensive care transport accompanied by a referring specialist or a specialist retrieval team. Intensive Care Med 2004;30(2):302–8.

[38] Flabouris A, Runciman WB, Levings B. Incidents during out-of-hospital patient transportation. Anaesth Intensive Care 2006;34(2):228–36.

[39] Lupton BA, Pendray MR. Regionalized neonatal emergency transport. Semin Neonatol 2004;9(2):125–33.

[40] Yun S, Faraj S, Sims HP. Contingent leadership and effectiveness of trauma resuscitation teams. J Appl Psychol 2005;90(6):1288–96.

[41] Fletcher G, Flin R, McGeorge P, et al. Anaesthetists' non-technical skills (ANTS): evaluation of a behavioural marker system. Br J Anaesth 2003;90(5):580–8.

[42] Hammond J. Simulation in critical care and trauma education and training. Curr Opin Crit Care 2004;10(5):325–9.

[43] Shapiro MJ, Morey JC, Small SD, et al. Simulation based teamwork training for emergency department staff: does it improve clinical team performance when added to an existing didactic teamwork curriculum? Qual Saf Health Care 2004;13(6):417–21.

[44] Lee SK, Pardo M, Gaba D, et al. Trauma assessment training with a patient simulator: a prospective randomized study. J Trauma 2003;55(4):651–7.

[45] Marshall RL, Smith JS, Gorman PJ, et al. Use of a human patient simulator in the development of resident trauma management skills. J Trauma 2001;51(1):17–21.

[46] Holcomb JB, Dumire RD, Crommett JW, et al. Evaluation of trauma team performance using an advanced human patient simulator for resuscitation training. J Trauma 2002;52(6): 1078–85.

[47] Hunt EA, Hohenhaus SM, Luo X, et al. Simulation of pediatric trauma stabilization in 35 North Carolina emergency departments: identification of targets for performance improvement. Pediatrics 2006;117(3):641–8.

ANESTHESIOLOGY
CLINICS

Anesthesiology Clin
25 (2007) 321–336

Virtual Worlds and Team Training

Parvati Dev, PhD[a],*, Patricia Youngblood, PhD[a],
W. LeRoy Heinrichs, MD, PhD[a],
Laura Kusumoto, MS[b]

[a]*SUMMIT, Stanford University School of Medicine, Stanford, CA 94305–5466, USA*
[b]*Forterra Systems, 1855 South Grant Road, 3rd Floor,
San Mateo, CA 94402, USA*

Medical education has increasingly adopted situated or experiential learning as an important component of medical training [1]. This training has taken the form of learning in a variety of simulated environments ranging from encounters with simulated patients to participation in team-based simulated medical activities [2,3]. A well-accepted simulation-based learning environment is one where a high-fidelity human simulator, an instrumented mannequin running a computational model of physiology and pharmacology, represents the patient, and a team of health care personnel manage the simulated medical case in a physical space representing an operating room or other hospital space. Virtual worlds provide the opportunity to replicate and extend this learning environment, supporting participation by multiple remotely located learners who access the virtual world simulation through the Internet, and manage the medical case as though they were together in a real space.

What is a virtual world?

The concept of a geometrically accurate, earth-size, virtual world, or "metaverse," was first articulated in a science-fiction novel [4]. It defines a virtual world as a computer-based, three-dimensional, spatially realistic, simulated environment intended to represent a real or fictional location [5]. The virtual world is operated on a server computer, or computer cluster, and users connect to the world from their local computers by the Internet.

This work was supported by the Wallenberg Foundation, the Telemedicine and Advanced Technology Research Center, and Adobe Systems.
* Corresponding author.
E-mail address: parvati@stanford.edu (P. Dev).

The virtual world resembles the real world, and has real world rules, such as distance, gravity, and the ability to move within the world. Buildings can be entered and explored. Objects may be interacted with, moved, or exchanged. In some virtual worlds, users can create new objects, creating new environments.

The virtual world may have multiple inhabitants, called "avatars," each selected from a library, and controlled by a person from their own computer. Avatars see each other in the world, and interact through voice or typed chat. Each person sees the world from the point-of-view of his or her avatar. The avatar's movement and action are controlled by the user's keyboard and mouse. Some inhabitants are controlled by computer programs, not live users, and have a predetermined suite of actions. These simulated inhabitants, called "robots," "robotars," or "nonplayer characters," may take many roles, such as participants in a crowd or a character with a limited set of required actions. Artificial intelligence programming may be added to these characters, increasing their capabilities, a factor that is important in medical virtual worlds.

Some virtual worlds have only one controllable character or avatar, and all other characters are computer controlled. Computer-controlled characters are preanimated, with a limited set of behaviors or animations that are rendered in response to the learner's actions. Artificial intelligence may be used to increase the range of behaviors available to these computer-controlled characters. Many medical virtual worlds are single-player worlds where the learner is placed in a crisis situation and must make decisions to manage the medical problem [6]. In contrast, in multiplayer worlds, most characters are controlled by real people [7–12]. The animations may be limited but voice, or text chat, allow freeform interaction.

A multiperson virtual world is a persistent world that exists even when the user logs off. This is different from many games and simulation environments that are active only while the user interacts with them. A virtual world continues to evolve while the user is away. Meanwhile, other users who are logged in can interact, exchange information, and modify, create, or remove objects, while the first user is away. A virtual world represents an approximation to some aspects of the real world, and may be used as a reasonable facsimile of a variety of real medical locations, such as hospital wards and intensive care units.

For those familiar with networked games, such as Sims Online, in multiplayer medical virtual worlds, the setting might be a hospital or other site, and each Sim character would be controlled by a different person. If any person logged off, the other characters might continue to play and evolve the state of the world. If a character was the patient and was controlled by a medical model, then the patient's state would evolve over time.

Simulated, or virtual, worlds were developed first by the military. Technology for airplane flight simulation grew rapidly during and after World War II, and was used to train pilots in necessary skills before they operated the actual airplane. These systems included a detailed simulation of aircraft mechanics and a three-dimensional rendering of the virtual world as seen through the aircraft windows [13,14]. By the 1980s, multiple such simulations were being linked, within one large three-dimensional virtual space, to support team learning in war games. Through these developments, considerable technologic expertise was developed both in the modeling and rendering of three-dimensional worlds and in real-time communication over networks [1].

At the same time, there was a grass-roots effort, mostly in academia, to make games available on the computer. Games that linked players over the network drew their inspiration from the popular Dungeons and Dragons board game. A multiuser dungeon or domain or dimension (MUD) is a multiplayer computer game that includes fantasy role-playing, battles, and social chat [15,16]. The game is text-based. Players read descriptions of rooms, objects, events, and other characters, and they interact with the surrounding space and each other through typed, English-like commands. MUD object-oriented (MOO), an extension of MUDs, even allowed players to extend the world themselves, adding objects and spaces to customize their virtual world. MOOs proliferated as educational tools, particularly in teaching writing and composition, as students used descriptive text to build new rooms and create new behaviors for objects in their game. MOO technology and game principles were influential in the subsequent development of graphical virtual worlds.

As the Internet became widely available, and as graphics capability improved, text-based networked games evolved into rich visual worlds, with realistic-looking characters and objects (usually weapons). These massively multiplayer online role-playing games shared some basic characteristics, derived from MOOs. The players moved in a three-dimensional world. Game play included quests, monsters, and loot. A point system was reflected in character development and levels of play. An associated economy existed for trade in weapons and tools. Social organization emerged, with guilds for collaborative action against enemies.

Multiplayer social worlds were an outgrowth of multiplayer game worlds [17,18]. A key capability of these social worlds is the creation of new objects by the user. The ability to personalize one's own character, and any virtual space that one has purchased, has allowed dramatic expansion of the number of activities available in these worlds. From three-dimensional chat rooms these worlds have evolved into spaces with many of the activities of the real world. Businesses have created virtual stores just as they created virtual store-fronts on the World Wide Web [19]. News organizations have virtual offices and reporters in these worlds [20,21].

The technology of online video games combined with the story telling experience of cinema were perceived as a rich source for fulfilling the training needs of the US Army. The potential of this confluence was demonstrated in an emotionally charged game scenario of an army lieutenant on a virtual Bosnian street, facing a complex decision-making situation [22]. Another army training game, America's Army, about training a soldier through simulated combat missions, was developed as a recruiting tool for the Army, and has since been developed into a series of games for actual soldier training [23,24]. This use of game technology for serious learning became an impetus for similar development in many other areas, including medicine.

Today there are many multiplayer "game engines" available. A game engine is the core software of a computer game. It provides rendering of two- or three-dimensional graphics of the world and its avatars. It may also compute the physics of gravity and of collisions in the world, the spatialization of sound, and any rules of interaction between avatars and with objects. Customizable engines include scripting languages to author objects and behaviors, and some provide the entire source code for full customization. The game engine also deals with all system issues, such as managing transmissions across the network, and synchronizing what is seen by all the players in the world.

Virtual worlds in medicine

Medical virtual worlds are specialized virtual worlds. The three-dimensional space includes buildings that represent a hospital, a clinic, or an emergency department. Objects include a range of medically relevant furniture, instruments, devices, and tools. The characters are clothed according to their relevant roles, such as a nurse, emergency medical technician, physician, patient, or bystander. The functions available to a character may also be restricted according to their role. A patient, for example, may not be able to connect an intravenous drip.

Army medical research has been a significant sponsor of new training methods to develop effective responses to mass casualty terrorist events, collectively categorized as chemical, biologic, radiologic-nuclear, and explosive (CBRNE) incidents [25]. Virtual worlds, originally developed for training of military personnel deployed in Iraq, were repurposed to train military first responders to a CBRNE incident [26].

Some virtual worlds have their roots in team training for emergency medicine based on the high-fidelity human mannequin simulation. In these worlds, the mannequin is replaced by a computer-modeled patient, and the team member roles are played by learners or faculty logged in from their individual computers [27].

With the advent of virtual worlds, simulations have moved outside the medical environment of the hospital. Virtual worlds have been built to represent trauma and mass casualty in city buildings and on streets. Virtual worlds have also been extended to learners outside the conventional medical arena, such as high school students learning decision-making for cardiopulmonary resuscitation [28,29].

A new approach to virtual worlds is to provide an immersive environment where the learner is surrounded by the medical situation [30]. In this case, the three-dimensional world is projected onto screens surrounding the learner. The learner wears goggles that support stereographic viewing, increasing the sense of being in a three-dimensional space. In the project cited [30], the learner is the only inhabitant in the world. Extending the capability to support both real and virtual participants is a challenging advance.

The scenario

Development of a virtual medical world must be preceded by the selection of the learning goals and, consequently, the scenario to be modeled. Fig. 1 shows the many parallel events that occur during a CBRNE incident. Only selected events in the timeline are simulated: the setup of the triage area, the triage process for the victims of the blast, and the transportation of the victims. The only part of the world to be simulated is in the immediate vicinity of the blast.

The world

For the example mentioned previously, a city building (a bank) and other building facades on the street are modeled in a three-dimensional world. Conventional graphics programs for three-dimensional objects can be used. The objects, such as buildings, are imported into the world and positioned according to the internal spatial coordinates in the world. The geometric extent of the world differs for each virtual world, with some being of the same size and shape of the Earth.

Objects necessary to the exercise are also modeled in a three-dimensional design program, and placed in the world. For a first responder exercise, these may include a drivable ambulance, a gurney, a decontamination tent, a Geiger counter, a basic aid kit, uniforms for the characters, and other objects. The number of such objects may be infinite or it may be finite, representing a limited resource.

An interactive object, such as a drivable ambulance, has not only a three-dimensional graphic appearance, but also various behaviors. It can move (ie, be driven) using keyboard and mouse controls. It can contain a driver, a passenger, and a gurney with a patient (Fig. 2). When it moves, these characters also are moved along. Similarly, a vital signs monitor, when connected to a patient, receives numeric data from the patient's medical model and displays them on a simulated screen. Each behavior is generated by a segment of computer code that is triggered by an action, such as a keystroke, or by an action of another character in the virtual world.

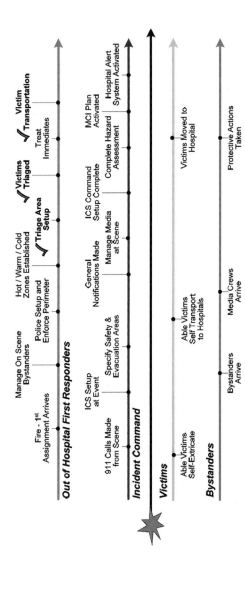

Fig. 1. Timeline of a bomb blast incident. The star icon indicates the time of the explosion. Time progresses to the right. First responders respond to a call from incident command. Victims transport themselves or are moved to the hospital. Bystanders also arrive and add to the confusion. Events with a check mark are selected for the simulation.

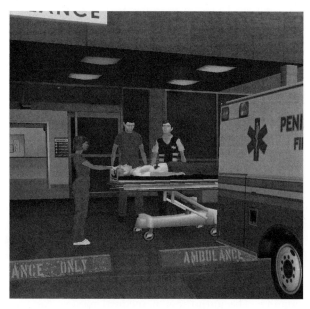

Fig. 2. Three avatars, representing emergency medical technician and the hospital staff, manage a patient on a gurney. The patient was delivered to this location by the ambulance visible.

Avatars

Avatars are three-dimensional graphic renditions of people. An avatar's movement, gestures, and actions are controlled by the user. Actions are created as animations in a three-dimensional animation program, imported into the world, and triggered by user controls. In some virtual world systems in which the avatar mechanics are controlled by a physics model, certain actions, such as the dynamic response to a collision, are generated by the model and do not need to be preanimated.

Conversational interaction between avatars may be through text chat in simpler worlds, and through voice in other worlds. Good voice interaction adds greatly to the immediacy and realism of the world, but poor audio quality can detract significantly from the user experience. For voice interaction, the user wears a headset with a microphone to reduce potential audio problems, such as echo. When learners are colocated in one room, headsets also give some audio isolation.

Medical models

Avatars, or computer-controlled characters, that represent patients require physiologic attributes and vital signs. They may also exhibit an evolution of their physiology over time, and the ability to respond to medical care. These characteristics are termed the "medical model" of the character.

Medical models, in the computer, may take many forms. One approach is a mathematical modeling approach, in which selected aspects of the physiology are represented through interacting equations, with parameters that respond to stimuli [31–33]. These models can have from a dozen to hundreds of equations and can represent physiology and pharmacology in great detail. Model equations and parameters are developed through extensive analysis of the literature and through carefully selected experiments. The validity of a model may be difficult to establish, and modifying a complex model may be very difficult for any except the original modeler.

A second approach to medical models is a rule-based approach. Rule-based medical models provide a great deal of flexibility but require detailed description of each possible interplay between the parameters of a scenario. Rule-based models can be developed quickly for simple medical situations but rapidly become intractable as medical complexity increases. With appropriate authoring languages, rules for each model can be developed with minimal programming. The authoring of medical models for virtual worlds, however, is still in its infancy [34].

When simulating a dirty bomb attack on a public building, a range of injury profiles is created. This causes the hospital triage team to generate a variety of immediacy classifications, thus stimulating the emergency department treatment areas with sufficient number and variety of cases to surface their need to work as a team and manage critical resources, such as beds and blood supplies. Example cases include men and women of varying ages and conditions receiving such injuries as lacerations, compound fractures, pneumothorax, major pelvic trauma, bruising, head injury, and liver lacerations. Each patient case describes the patient overall (gender, age, pre-existing medical conditions); injuries caused by the disaster; the diagnoses and treatments that an expert team might make; and the responses the patient will show if properly treated in time, or not. Each case is programmed using the medical model. The model's state evolves over time, and can be modified through various therapeutic procedures, such as appropriate life-support procedures or medications. In the absence of remediation, severely impaired patients succumb to asphyxiation, hemorrhage, or other problems.

Physiologic attributes must be presented in a visual or other form for other avatars to see, use, and react to this information. For example, symptoms may be presented as spoken words, text, images, or representations on the three-dimensional avatar. Tradeoffs must be made between the most "realistic" presentation, the computational impact of a particular style of presentation, whether the presentation is sufficient for meeting learning objectives, and the cost of development. For example, examining a patient's pupil response is very important, but rendering many views of the pupil on the avatar is expensive. Instead an illustration is displayed showing the state of the pupil as determined in the medical model. Bleeding and bruising cannot be relegated to pictures that are separate from the avatar, however, so bleeding and bruising are depicted on the three-dimensional avatar.

Learning objectives

In a typical trauma or CBRNE training incident, there can be many learning objectives. When using multiplayer virtual worlds, training is focused most appropriately on the interaction between the participants in their role as team members. Typically, the virtual world is not appropriate for training in procedural skills, such as insertion of an intravenous cannula, which is learned better individually using other methods. Learning objectives can be selected based on the need to train for leadership, communication, resource management, professionalism, or other aspects of team training.

Training method

The training method used in these virtual worlds is simulation-based learning with "after-action review," or "debriefing." In this training approach, individual learners control avatars in a simulated three-dimensional world where a CBRNE event has occurred. Learners enter the world from geographically dispersed locations by logging onto the training system's Web site and an instructor leads the exercise. During the exercise, learners interact with each other and victims, according to the specific protocols that they have learned previously. Once complete, the instructor uses observations made during the scenario to conduct an after-action review.

The style of training used for this research is based on experiential learning in which learners participate in a shared learning experience. Once the exercise is complete, they work with the instructor or facilitator, aided by videos captured during the exercise, to understand how they might improve their performance in the next iteration of the training scenario. To lead this style of training, the instructor's role is to brief the trainees at the beginning of the exercise to introduce them to the rules of the game, and to observe and listen to the interactions that occur during the scenario. After the scenario has ended, the instructor leads a follow-up discussion with the learners to elicit from them what worked well and what they may have done differently.

Assessment

To facilitate and standardize trainee debriefing, it is useful to create a score sheet for items to be measured, and to train all raters on the use of the score sheet. Clear examples should be provided of behaviors that should be scored as average, below average, or above average. An example is shown later of a score sheet and rating scale developed for use by the facilitator, based on existing score sheets for crisis resource management in emergency medicine.

Evaluation

Medical virtual worlds are still in their infancy, and most have not yet been evaluated for their efficacy in training or their ability to engage the learner. An early virtual world, SimTech, was built by the authors to emulate mannequin-based, human patient simulation capability [35]. A team of four medical avatars, one of whom was a student or resident, managed a series of trauma cases in a virtual emergency room. The other three avatars were played by team members and represented a nurse and other support personnel.

Each patient was a computer-controlled character with a simple rule-based medical model. The patient presented with a trauma situation, such as an 18-year-old boy who fell off a bicycle and sustained internal injuries because of impact with the handle bar. If no action is taken, the medical model causes the patient's physiology to evolve and worsen. Appropriate action, such as administering oxygen or inserting the appropriate intravenous catheters, stabilizes the patient, who can then be admitted to the hospital for further care (Figs. 3 and 4).

The learners were fourth-year medical students or first-year residents, all of whom had been through a course for advanced trauma life support. After a training session, each team was given a pretest trauma case, followed by four learning cases, then a posttest case. Each learning case was followed by a debriefing session where team members and the learner discussed the actions taken.

For comparison, a comparable group was trained using the Human Patient Simulator mannequin in a traditional simulation setting. They were also given training, followed by a pretest case, four learning cases, and a posttest case. The same cases were used in both the environments.

Learners were rated using a scale shown in Boxes 1 and 2, based on the Emergency Medicine Crisis Resource Management scale previously developed by one of the team members for use in mannequin-based training. Multiple raters were used and the interrater reliability was high.

Learners in the virtual world showed significant improvement in performance between pretest and posttest cases (Fig. 5). During the debriefing sessions, they indicated that the virtual world simulation stimulated their recollection of advanced trauma life support procedures leading to improvements with each case. Learners using the Human Patient Simulator also showed significant improvement in performance between pre-test and post-test cases, indicating the system's learning efficacy. Interestingly, there

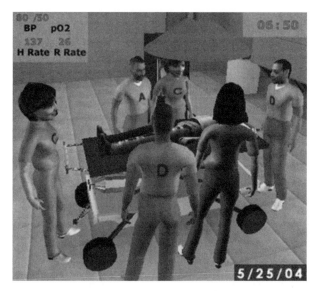

Fig. 3. The emergency department team, represented by their avatars, manages the computer-controlled patient on the gurney.

was no significant difference in performance between the two systems, indicating that, for the basic trauma cases selected, the virtual world was as effective for learning as the more traditional Human Patient Simulator [36].

Future developments

Virtual worlds have demonstrated promising results in medical team training in areas critical to patient safety and error reduction. The method

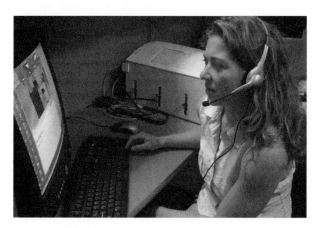

Fig. 4. A learner, speaking through a headset, controls her character with the mouse, and observes the actions of the team members in the world depicted on her computer screen.

Box 1. Rating scale of team performance

Items to be measured (rating from 1 to 5)
Knowledge of the environment
Anticipation of and planning for potential problems
Assumption of leadership role
Communication with other team members
Distribution of workload, delegation of responsibility
Attention allocation
Use of information
Use of resources
Recognition of limitations
Professional behavior, interpersonal skills
Overall team leadership skills

---

1 = not acceptable
5 = excellent

---

is being extended to the training of multiple simultaneous teams managing a stream of patients in a simulation of a large-scale disaster. The Virtual Emergency Department has been expanded to a multibay department, with adjacent related facilities, such as an ambulance bay, a decontamination tent, reception area, and an emergency triage area. Other applications are also being evaluated, in particular the training of high school students in group management of crises involving the collapse of a person through fainting, choking, or a heart attack, with the associated communication and decision-making challenges (Fig. 6).

An important area of research is the development and evaluation of complex medical models. Model complexity should be determined by the requirements of the learning objectives. These models need to be evaluated for construct and content validity for these learning objectives. Model types,

---

Box 2. Scoring an item: attention allocation

Average: Pays attention to the changes in the vital signs on the monitors, and to the patient
Below: Focuses on only one thing, like the fracture, or one vital sign
Above: Pays attention to all vital signs on the monitors, and the patient himself or herself, and also to all team members to make sure they are performing appropriately

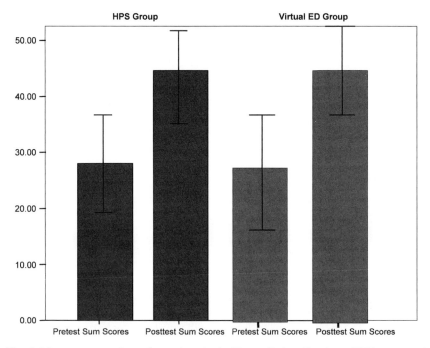

Fig. 5. Mean scores are shown for students in the Human Patient Simulator (HPS) group and in the Virtual Emergency Department (ED) group. Significant and comparable improvement is displayed by both groups between pretest and posttest cases.

such as rule-based and mathematical models, should be studied to determine their areas of application. It is possible that simple rule-based models may be optimal for the simulation of a large number of patients converging on an emergency department in a crisis, whereas the patients actually in the emergency room bay may need to be simulated with higher fidelity using a mathematical model.

Assessment methods have been developed for individual performance, with some metrics also available for team performance. As multiple simultaneous teams interact in a virtual world, new assessment tools need to be developed both for team performance and for the performance of the entire unit. Current methods rely mostly on check lists and observer rating of team members. Because these simulations involve a large number of simultaneous learners, observer-based rating methods need to be augmented with other objective, automated measurement tools.

Hybrid simulations, involving real and virtual components, are on the horizon [37]. The three-dimensional environment is presented in an immersive virtual presentation using large displays surrounding the learner. The learner is physically present and may interact with a physical mannequin representing the patient. Alternatively, the learner may use a procedure

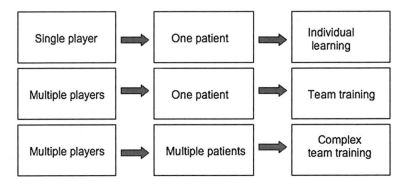

Fig. 6. A matrix of the learning possibilities in different types of virtual worlds. A virtual world may have one or more characters controlled by real players. Other characters, if present, are computer-controlled. The players manage one or more simultaneously available patients. Managing multiple patients increases the complexity of the learning situation. It also increases the complexity of the performance metrics.

simulator while surrounded by a virtual environment. Single-person simulations, combining real and immersive virtual environments, have been demonstrated. The next step is to integrate the multiplayer virtual world into the immersive virtual environment, with the real and the avatar characters interacting and communicating in the scenario.

Another important link between real and virtual worlds is when data from real sensors feed into the virtual world, driving monitors and even medical models. A first step is being planned where a cardiopulmonary resuscitation mannequin is instrumented, and a student interacting with it sees himself or herself in the virtual world administering cardiopulmonary resuscitation to a virtual patient.

The opportunities are immense for the use of virtual worlds in training for optimal performance and error reduction. Virtual environments are not restricted to in-hospital environments. Training settings can be a city street, a crowded train, a nuclear facility, or an elementary school, all places where it is very difficult to run a physical training exercise. Further, the ability for each person to enter a virtual world from anywhere in the real world makes it possible to train multidisciplinary teams well before they are actually needed to get together in a disaster location. Considerable research is needed on the technology, the pedagogic methods, and the assessment tools, but the promise of this powerful new tool is extremely attractive.

References

[1] Singhal S, Zyda M. Networked virtual environments: design and implementation. Addison-Wesley Professional; 1999.
[2] Gaba DM. The future vision of simulation in health care. Qual Saf Health Care 2004; 13(Suppl 1):i2–10.

[3] Salas E, Burke CS, Cannon-Bowers JA. What we know about designing and delivering team training: tips and guidelines. In: Kraiger K, editor. Creating, implementing, and managing effective training and development: state-of-the-art lessons for practice. San Francisco (CA): Jossey-Bass; 2002.

[4] Stephenson N. Snow crash. Spectra; 1992.

[5] Wikipedia. Virtual world. Available at: http://en.wikipedia.org/wiki/Virtual_world. Accessed March 3, 2007.

[6] Jain R. Taking the pulse!! of medical training. Business week online. April 10, 2006, Available at: http://www.businessweek.com/innovate/content/apr2006/id20060410_051875.htm. Accessed March 19, 2007.

[7] Wladawsky-Berger I. Transforming business through virtual worlds capabilities—it's Déjà Vu all over again. Available at: http://irvingwb.typepad.com/blog/2006/09/transforming_bu.html. Accessed March 3, 2007.

[8] Tiffany L. Starting a second life business. Available at: http://www.msnbc.msn.com/id/17280460/. Accessed March 3, 2007.

[9] Loftus T. Virtual world teaches real-world skills. Available at: http://www.msnbc.msn.com/id/7012645/. Accessed Mar 3, 2007. (autism)

[10] Boyle A. Virtual worlds offer real-world healing. Available at: http://www.msnbc.msn.com/id/17286291/wid/11915829/. Accessed March 3, 2007. (not multiperson).

[11] Skeen D. Yoicks! It's another virtual world. Available at: http://www.theage.com.au/news/biztech/yoicks-its-another-virtual-world/2007/02/26/1172338546871.html. Accessed March 3, 2007.

[12] Konrad R. IBM launches push into virtual world. AP News report. Available at: http://www.msnbc.msn.com/id/16545338/. Accessed March 3, 2007.

[13] Rolfe JM, Staples KJ. Flight simulation. Cambridge University Press; 1988.

[14] Moore K. A brief history of aircraft flight simulation. Available at: http://homepage.ntlworld.com/bleep/SimHist1.html. Accessed January 1, 2007.

[15] Busey A, Poirier J. Secrets of the mud wizards: playing and programming muds, moos, mucks, and other internet role-playing games. Sams; 1995.

[16] National Research Council Report. Modeling and simulation: linking entertainment and defense. Washington, DC: National Academy Press; 1997.

[17] Costa D. Virtual worlds. PC Magazine, vol. 28, no. 19. October 28, 2003. Available at: http://www.pcmag.com/article2/0,1759,1306175,00.asp. Accessed March 3, 2007.

[18] Foster AL. The avatars of research: students and professors join popular virtual worlds like second life to study the real-world interactions they represent. The Chronicle of Higher Education, September 30, 2005. Available at: http://chronicle.com/weekly/v52/i06/06a03501.htm. Accessed March 3, 2007.

[19] Kirkpatrick S. It's not a game. The 3-D online experience Second Life is a hit with users. IBM's Sam Palmisano and other tech leaders think it could also be a gold mine. Fortune Magazine.vol. 155, no. 2. February 5, 2007. Available at: http://money.cnn.com/magazines/fortune/fortune_archive/2007/02/05/8399120/index.htm. Accessed March 3, 2007.

[20] Wired. Wired in second life. Wired Magazine, October 10, 2006. Available at: http://www.wired.com/wired/archive/14.10/slwired.html. Accessed March 3, 2007.

[21] Stevens V. Second life and online collaboration through peer to peer distributed learning networks. To be presented at METSMaC Conference, March 17-19, 2007, Abu Dhabi. Available at: http://www.homestead.com/prosites-vstevens/files/efi/papers/metsmac/metsmac_secondlife.htm. Accessed March 3, 2007.

[22] Rickel J, Gratch J, Marsella S, et al. Steve goes to Bosnia: towards a new generation of virtual humans for interactive experiences. AAAI Spring Symposium on Artificial Intelligence and Interactive Entertainment. Stanford University (CA), March 2001.

[23] America's army: special forces. Available at: http://www.americasarmy.com/. Accessed January 1, 2007.

[24] Zyda M. Weapons of mass distraction–America's army recruits for the Real War. Presented at the State of Play Conference, held at the New York Law School. Available: http://gamepipe.usc.edu/≈;zyda/presentations/Games&LawTalk-15Nov2003.pdf. (large file), 2003.

[25] Marks R. Defining America's brave new world. Cambridge Review of International Affairs 2002;15(No 2):329–43.

[26] Kaufman M, Dev P, Youngblood P. Application of multiplayer game technology to team based training of medical first responders. Orlando (FL): I/ITSEC; 2005.

[27] Youngblood P, Harter P, Srivastava S, et al. A virtual learning environment for team training in trauma management. Acad Emerg Med 2005;12:792–3.

[28] Youngblood P, Hedman L, Creutzfeld J, et al. Virtual worlds for teaching the new CPR to high school students. MMVR 2007.

[29] Srivastava S, Harter P, Youngblood P, et al. A web-based virtual 3D world for team training in trauma management. MMVR 2005.

[30] Lee CH, Liu A, Del Castillo S, et al. Towards an immersive virtual environment for medical team training. Presented at the Medicine Meets Virtual Reality. San Diego (CA). February 2007.

[31] Philip JH. GAS MAN: a pictorial and graphical simulation for teaching anesthesia uptake and distribution [abstract]. Atlanta (GA): ASA, Anesthesiology. vol. 59;A471:1983.

[32] Garfield JM, Paskin S, Philip JH. An evaluation of the effectiveness of a computer simulation of anaesthetic uptake and distribution as a teaching tool. Med Educ 1989;23:457–62.

[33] Gaba DM, DeAnda A. A comprehensive anesthesia simulation environment: re-creating the operating room for research and training. Anesthesiology 1988;69:387–94.

[34] Dev P, Heinrichs WL, Youngblood P, et al. Virtual patient model for multi-person virtual medical environments, submitted to the Annual Conference of the American Medical Informatics Association, November, 2007.

[35] SimTech. Available at: http://simtech.stanford.edu/. Accessed March 7, 2007.

[36] Youngblood P, Srivastava S, Harter P, et al. Validation of a web-based VR simulation for training trauma teams. MMVR 2005.

[37] Lee CH, Liu A, Del Castillo S, et al. Towards an immersive virtual environment for medical team training. Presented at the Medicine Meets Virtual Reality, February 2007. Available at: http://www.simcen.org/pdf/lee_mmvr07%20ver%202.pdf. Accessed March 3, 2007.

ANESTHESIOLOGY
CLINICS

ELSEVIER
SAUNDERS

Anesthesiology Clin
25 (2007) 337–348

Virtual Reality Simulations

P. Pat Banerjee, PhD[a,b,c,]*, Cristian J. Luciano, MS[d], Silvio Rizzi, MS[d]

[a]*Department of Mechanical and Industrial Engineering (M/C 251), University of Illinois-Chicago, 3029 Engineering Research Facility, 842 West Taylor Street, Chicago, IL 60607, USA*
[b]*Department of Computer Science, University of Illinois-Chicago, 3029 Engineering Research Facility, 842 West Taylor Street, Chicago, IL 60607, USA*
[c]*Department of Bioengineering, University of Illinois-Chicago, 3029 Engineering Research Facility, 842 West Taylor Street, Chicago, IL 60607, USA*
[d]*Department of Mechanical and Industrial Engineering, University of Illinois-Chicago, 1024 Engineering Research Facility, 842 West Taylor Street, Chicago, IL 60607, USA*

Earlier reviews on applications of virtual reality (VR) in anesthesia [1] cover many aspects of VR technology, as it evolved, and make many insightful comments about its potential. According to Burt [1], the advantages include simulating critical events at no risk to the patient; the ability to repeat, halt, record, replay and reproduce, critique, and objectively evaluate control of independent or multiple variables; and high-fidelity execution. Although most of Burt's [1] observations have been subsequently well researched, it is the high-fidelity execution that is still in its infancy. Burt [1] criticizes the low resolution of head-mounted display for VR and emphasizes the need to replace it with higher-resolution monitor screens. Subsequent approaches, such as those of Blezek and colleagues [2] in 2000, have continued with the use of head-mounted displays in their VR simulation of regional anesthesia for training of residents at Mayo Clinic in Rochester, Minnesota. Blezek and colleagues [2] combined VR with haptics, following work done at Ohio State University [3,4], on a force-feedback model for an epidural needle insertion simulator. This epidural block simulator incorporates a one degree of freedom force feedback device, and visualization through stereo glasses using a desktop computer monitor. Blezek and colleagues [2] use PHANToM force feedback device [5], a head-mounted stereo display, and a magnetic tracking system for tracking the user's head. The data are obtained after segmenting volumetric data from

---

* Corresponding author.
E-mail address: banerjee@uic.edu (P.P. Banerjee).

National Library of Medicine's visible human male CT datasets. They perform a series of biomechanical needle-force experiments on unembalmed male cadavers within 72 hours of death. The instrumented needle has been used to perform the standard retrocrural celiac plexus block procedure several times for each cadaver. For each needle insertion, the position of the needle has been obtained from a tracking system. Using force transducer voltage data, needle force versus penetration depth graphs have been drawn. Needle force has been calculated by converting force cell voltages from volt to Newton. Penetration distance has been determined by using a thresholding process on the collected force data. The point at which the needle encountered the skin surface is clearly identifiable in the collected force data. By a detailed analysis of all collected datasets, a mathematical model of needle force has been developed. The force model has been implemented using the C++ programming language within the framework of the PHANToM software development environment (SensAble Technologies, Woburn, Massachusetts). To calculate haptic feedback forces, a CT dataset is used to calculate skin intersection positions, forces within the soft tissue, and intersection with bony structures.

A survey of approximately 100 practicing anesthesiologists included the following four questions: (1) What effect would the VR training system have on resident teaching? (2) If a patient with difficult anatomy presented, would I first rehearse the procedure on the simulator? (3) What is the most important aspect of regional anesthesia? and (4) What is the second most important aspect of regional anesthesia? Blezek and colleagues [2] obtained the answers outlined in Table 1.

Eason [6] at East Tennessee State University reviewed AccuTouch (Immersion Medical, Gaithersburg, Maryland), a computerized VR bronchoscopy simulator. The device consists of a proxy flexible bronchoscope, a robotic interface device with an orifice, a computer monitor, and simulation software. The operator inserts the bronchoscope into the interface and views a VR anatomic representation of the airway on the computer monitor. The anatomy is generated from data derived from the dataset of the three-dimensional computer-generated model of the airway from the National Library of Medicine's Visible Human project. Rowe and Cohen [7], from Children's Hospital Oakland and the University of California at San Francisco, experimentally test the hypothesis that the AccuTouch is an effective way to teach clinicians the psychomotor skills necessary for fiberoptic intubation (FOI) of the trachea of a pediatric patient. Pediatric residents with no prior experience in FOI were studied. Residents performed FOI on children undergoing general anesthesia. Tapes of these intubations were analyzed for time to visualization of the carina and number of times that the bronchoscope tip hit the mucosa. Residents then studied an average of 17 cases, and spent 39 minutes on the simulator. Time to completion of successful intubation with a bronchoscope was reduced from 5.15 to 0.88 minutes. The number of times that the tip of the bronchoscope hit the mucosa was

Table 1
Survey responses

(a) What effect would the VR training system have on resident teaching?	
Answer	Percentage
Greatly enhance	64
Marginally enhance	34
No effect	2
Slightly detrimental	0
Greatly detrimental	0
(b) If a patient with difficult anatomy presented, would I first rehearse the procedure on the simulator?	
Every time	42
Sometimes	55
Rarely	4
Never	0
(c) What is the most important aspect of regional anesthesia?	
Visualizing the anatomy	65
Feel of the needle	22
Procedure and workflow	9
Emergency procedures	4
(d) What is the second most important aspect of regional anesthesia?	
Visualizing the anatomy	28
Feel of the needle	50
Procedure and workflow	13
Emergency procedures	9

reduced from 21.4 to 0.19 minutes. The percent of time viewing the channel of the airway increased from 58.5% to 80.4%.

Goldmann and Steinfeldt [8] at Philipps University, Marburg, Germany, also studied acquisition of basic AccuTouch FOI skill using a similar hypothesis. The measurements included time to intubation before and after a 4-day training period using an adult VR FOI scenario and time to intubation using a fresh human cadaver 2 weeks after the training experience. Residents were able significantly to improve time to intubation in the VR scenario (114 versus 75 seconds). Novices differed from experienced attending anesthesiologists in time to intubation in the VR scenario, before but not after training (114 versus 79 seconds compared with 75 versus 72 seconds). Novices who had been trained with the simulator performed significantly faster in the cadaver than novices who had not (24 versus 86 seconds). Furthermore, there was no difference in time to intubation in the cadaver between trained novices and experienced attending anesthesiologists (24 versus 23 seconds). They concluded that use of a VR airway simulator enables anesthesia residents to acquire basic FOI skills comparable with those of experienced anesthesiologists in a human cadaver.

Other studies of relevance to anesthesiology include Satava [9], who performed a review of VR for medical applications, and Gaba [10], who presented the overall significance of simulation-based crisis resource management training for trauma care. The term "part task" simulation is frequently used by the US Department of Defense to signify that VR simulations are most useful when used to simulate portions of surgical tasks that involve difficult psychomotor skills rather than entire sets of surgical tasks.

VR and haptic technologies used in anesthesiology have one or more of the following limitations: (1) low resolution or low visual acuity, (2) highly obtrusive head-mounted display, and (3) lack of robust haptics-graphics collocation. How to overcome these technologic limitations is addressed in subsequent sections.

Virtual reality and on-demand high-fidelity simulation

According to David C. Leach, Executive Director of the Accreditation Council for Graduate Medical Education, simulation will be part of the redesign of graduate medical education [11]. It is important to understand some of the technical underpinnings of simulation because it will directly impact expensive investment decisions. High-fidelity simulators involve more sophisticated use of VR than the rudimentary form examined in the previous section. The ability to develop patient-specific situations on-demand is a key goal of VR-based high-fidelity simulators. Given the enormous variation in human anatomy and the substantial investment in building a simulation facility, the on-demand approach is likely to prevent a simulator from rapid obsolescence [12]. A historical perspective of VR and haptic technologies helps one understand its contribution to and potential for high-fidelity simulators.

In 1992, a room-sized four-walled projection-based three-dimensional VR system known as CAVE (CAVE Automatic Virtual Environment) was invented at the University of Illinois at Chicago (UIC) [13]. The popular CAVE technology has undergone a number of enhancements for over a decade to overcome its comparatively low-resolution graphics, resulting in low visual acuity and lack of brightness. The most recent manifestation of the CAVE in 2006 at Iowa State University, known as the 100-megapixel resolution six-walled C6 [14], has the technologic capability for developing real life-sized high-fidelity three-dimensional VR mannequins. The more than $4 million price tag for a Hewlett-Packard computer featuring 96 graphics processing units, 24 Sony digital projectors, an eight-channel audio system, and ultrasonic motion tracking, however, makes the technology quite expensive for simulators in the near future. More extensive testing on the use of the technology also needs to be conducted to make it ready for developing high-fidelity life-sized simulators.

Starting in 1994, there has been a parallel effort underway at UIC, known as ImmersaDesk [15], to develop more cost-effective large desktop displays. The first such system was built for the National Institute of Standards and Technology in 1995. The latest manifestation, known as ImmersaDesk4, is built from two Apple 30-in, 2560 × 1600, LCD panels mounted with quarter-wave plates in front of the LCD panels to achieve circular polarization (Fig. 1). The LCD panels are bisected by a half-silvered mirror, which

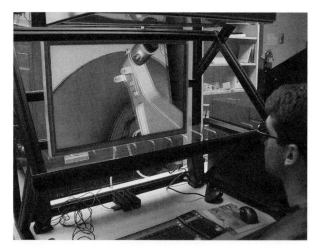

Fig. 1. The ImmersaDesk4 system is suitable for high-fidelity desktop simulations. (*Courtesy of* ImmersiveTouch, Chicago, IL.)

reverses the polarization of the top LCD panel. An optional three-dimensional position and orientation tracking system can be attached to allow the computer graphics to project the correct viewer-centered stereoscopic imagery based on the user's head position and orientation. A number of companies, such as Planar Systems [16], have commercialized previous generations of this technology. The ImmersaDesk technology has been used to create a collocated VR and haptic technology known as the Personal Augmented Reality Immersive System (PARIS). [17,18], more details of which are presented in the next section.

ImmersiveTouch technology

The ImmersaDesk, like the CAVE, suffers from occlusion of the image by the hand or wand [15]. This occlusion is common to all rear-projected displays. When a virtual object is within arms length it is possible to place the arm behind the virtual object, but the arm always appears in front of the virtual object because the virtual object is projected on the screen. This situation often breaks the visual illusion, which is key for a VR experience. As a way to avoid this problem, Johnson and colleagues [17] at UIC designed PARIS, an ImmersaDesk-sized display that uses two mirrors to fold the optics, a translucent rear projection screen, and a half-silvered mirror to create a projection-based augmented reality display on a desktop. The projector is used to illuminate the translucent screen that sits above the user. The user, sitting at the desk, works with his or her hands below the mirror, allowing the use of a keyboard and mouse on the desktop, manipulating virtual objects using the traditional wand or gloves. The placement of the components, their relationship to the physical design, and their ergonomic affect on the user are critical. Although Johnson and colleagues [17] prefer to use a flat panel display, such as a plasma panel or an LCD panel, the technology is not robust enough to provide a large stereo display. PARIS is a projection-based augmented reality system that uses two mirrors to fold the optics and a translucent black rear-projection screen illuminated by a Christie Mirage 2000 stereo DLP projector. The user looks through the half-silvered mirror that reflects the image projected onto the horizontal screen located above the user's head. The screen is positioned outside the user's field of view, such that only the reflected image is viewable by the user looking at the virtual projection plane. This is important; because the mirror is translucent, the brightness of the image projected on the screen is higher than the brightness of the image reflected by the mirror. Otherwise, the screen would easily distract the user.

The essential idea behind haptic augmented reality systems is to keep the collocation of the graphic representation and the haptic feedback of the virtual object. To maintain certain realistic eye-hand coordination, the user has to see and touch the same three-dimensional point in the virtual environment. In PARIS, a head tracking system handled by a dedicated networked tracking personal computer enhances this collocation. The head position and orientation is continuously sent to the rendering personal computer over the network to display a viewer-centered perspective. This configuration is similar in the CAVE and the ImmersaDesk. In PARIS, the tracking personal computer uses a pcBIRD (Ascension Technologies, Burlington, Vermont) for head and hand tracking. Despite a number of innovations, PARIS has technical barriers that prevent widespread surgical applications development. These limitations are addressed in ImmersiveTouch, described next.

The latest device, known as ImmersiveTouch (Fig. 2), has been quite successful in developing on-demand high-fidelity simulations. ImmersiveTouch is a patent-pending next-generation augmented VR technology invented by Banerjee and colleagues [19] at UIC. It is the first system that integrates a haptic device, with a head and hand tracking system, and a high-resolution and high pixel density stereoscopic display (see Fig. 2). Its ergonomic design provides a comfortable working volume in the space of a standard desktop. The haptic device is colocated with the three-dimensional graphics, giving the user a more realistic and natural means to manipulate and modify three-dimensional data in real time. The high-performance, multisensorial computer interface allows easy development of VR simulation and training applications that appeal to audio, visual, tactile, and kinesthetic stimuli.

ImmersiveTouch represents a complete hardware and software solution. The hardware integrates three-dimensional stereo visualization, force feedback, head and hand tracking, and three-dimensional audio. The software provides a unified applications programming interface to handle volume processing, graphics rendering, haptics rendering, three-dimensional audio feedback, interactive menus, and buttons. ImmersiveTouch is an evolutionary VR system resulting from the integration of a series of hardware

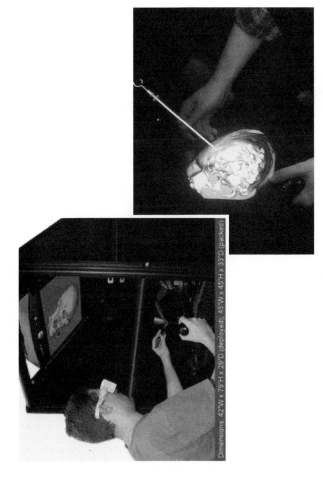

Fig. 2. ImmersiveTouch. Ventriculostomy simulation is depicted, showing the observer's view and the operator's view. (*Courtesy of* ImmersiveTouch, Chicago, IL.)

solutions to three-dimensional display issues and the development of a unique VR software platform (applications programming interface) drawing heavily on open-source software and databases.

ImmersiveTouch is based on open source software Coin (Open Inventor, Systems in Motion, Norway) for graphics rendering; Visualization Toolkit (VTK, Kitware, Clifton Park, New York) for volume processing; GHOST SDK and more recently OpenHaptics library (SenAble, Woburn, Massachusetts) for haptic rendering; pciBIRD API (Ascension Tech, Burlington, Vermont) for head and hand tracking; FLTK for the GUI and the OpenGL interface; and OpenAL for the three-dimensional audio. Ventriculostomy models for neurosurgical simulation content demonstration have been acquired from CT scans at the University of Illinois Medical Center and have been segmented using 3D Doctor (Able Software, Lexington, Massachusetts). A virtual model of a catheter from Medtronic Corporation has been developed. The eye model for cataract simulation has been developed by a contracted modeler. The three-dimensional teeth model has been obtained from Viewpoint (Digimation, Athens, Greece).

Off-the-shelf hardware components include a CRT monitor; a PHANToM haptic device; a dual-processor personal computer workstation; Crystal Eyes Stereo shutter glasses (Real D, Beverly Hills, California); and SpaceGrips hand controller (LaserAid, Los Gatos, California).

To understand the display hardware of the ImmersiveTouch simulator better, the following attributes for assessing augmented reality displays have been addressed:

- The created three-dimensional image allows the user's hands to be freely integrated with the virtual space and provide a natural means of interaction. Ideally, movement or placement of the user's head or hand should not occlude or interrupt the three-dimensional display.
- The user needs to be able to see and touch any three-dimensional point in the virtual environment at the same location in physical space to maintain realistic eye-hand coordination (haptics-graphics collocation). Essentially, the VR experience should be as close to real as possible.
- Visual acuity of the display needs to be close to perfect vision. Visual acuity for displays [20] is calculated as field of view (in degrees) x 1200/ display pixel resolution in the orientation of field of view.
- Viewer-centered perspective: Scene self-adjusts as viewer's perspective changes, just like in the real world.
- Size of workspace should be sufficient to allow full hand movement and interaction with the virtual three-dimensional image.
- Ability to read text shown in the image.
- Image refresh rates allow for smooth moving images, easy on the user's eyes.

No augmented VR graphic display system currently on the market has all of these attributes. The ImmersiveTouch simulator is significantly better

Table 2
Comparative features of various virtual reality and hepatic systems

Feature	PARIS™	Reachin™	SenseGraphics	ImmersiveTouch™
Display refresh rate	108Hz	120Hz	60Hz	100Hz
Pixel density	22 ppi	75 ppi	58 ppi	100 ppi
Visual acuity (20/20 = perfect)	20/113	20/33	20/82	20/24.75

The red lettering or red blocks indicate unacceptable range, brown or black lettering indicates borderline range, and blue lettering indicates acceptable range. Ppi, number of pixels per inch of display.

than any display hardware system (PARIS; Reachin, Stockholm, Sweden; and Sensegraphics, Kista Sweden) currently on the market as highlighted in Table 2. A feature summary is provided in Fig. 3.

A neurosurgical application of ImmersiveTouch is provided in the Appendix. A much broader effort is currently underway at UIC using the ImmersiveTouch simulator for different types of high-fidelity simulations. Eventually, a proposed UIC Medical Center Institute of Patient Safety Excellence will house many of these simulations.

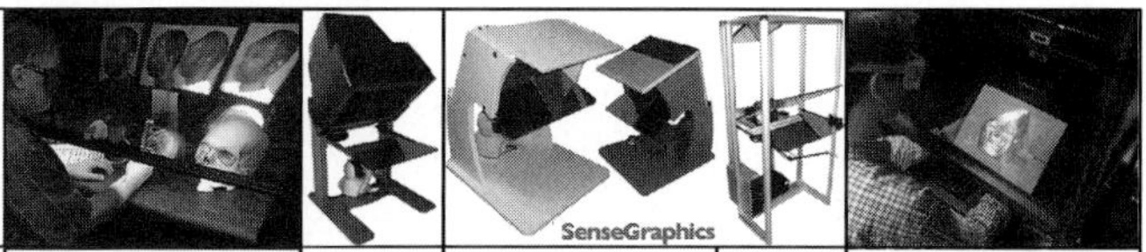

Feature	PARIS	Reachin Display	3D-MIW	3D-LIW	ImmersiveTouch
Display resolution	Regular	Regular	Low	Low	High
Pixel density & visual acuity	Low	Regular	Low	Low	High
Haptic and graphic volumes match	No	Yes	Yes	Yes	Yes
Head and hand tracking	Yes	No	No	No	Yes
Comfortable wide mirror	Yes	No	No	Yes	Yes
Only reflected image is viewable	Yes	No	Yes	Yes	Yes

Fig. 3. Comparative attributes of augmented VR graphic display systems currently on the market. (*Courtesy of* ImmersiveTouch, Chicago, IL.)

Summary

The goal of on-demand high-fidelity VR and haptically enabled simulations leads to three major advantages: (1) flexibility, (2) reusability, and (3) telemedicine compatibility. The simulator can be flexible enough to be able to handle a variety of clinical situations, its building blocks are reusable, and because the simulator operates in the VR and haptic domains, its contents can be transmitted and downloaded through the Internet, thereby promoting telemedical techniques.

Appendix

As a demonstration of an on-demand high-fidelity procedure simulation using ImmersiveTouch, an example from neurosurgery is presented to provide more insight. Similar procedures in other specialties including anesthesiology are being considered. Ventriculostomy is a neurosurgical procedure that consists of the insertion of a catheter into the ventricles of the brain for relieving intracranial pressure. A distinct "popping" sensation is felt as the catheter enters the ventricles. Early low-fidelity ventriculostomy simulators provided some basic audiovisual feedback to simulate the procedure, displaying a three-dimensional virtual model of a human head. Without any tactile feedback, the usefulness of such simulators was very limited. The first-generation haptic ventriculostomy simulators incorporated a haptic device to generate a virtual resistance and "give" on ventricular entry. Haptic feedback offers simulated resistance and relaxation with passage of a virtual three-dimensional ventriculostomy catheter through the brain parenchyma into the ventricle. Although this created considerable excitement as a novelty device for cannulating ventricles, its usefulness for teaching and measuring neurosurgical expertise was still very limited. Lack of crucial high-fidelity features led to poor collocation between the haptic device stylus held by the surgeon and the visual representation of the virtual catheter, and the lack of a correct viewer-centered perspective created enormous confusion for the neurosurgeons who diverted their attention from the actual ventriculostomy procedure to overcoming the limitations of the simulator. The ImmersiveTouch technology, which gives birth to a second-generation haptic ventriculostomy simulator, succeeds over the major first-generation limitations by introducing a head and hand tracking system and a high-resolution high visual acuity stereoscopic display to enhance the perception and realism of the virtual ventriculostomy (Fig. 4) [21].

A recent study, which is currently undergoing neurosurgical journal publication review, compares the performance of 78 neurosurgical fellows and residents for accuracy of ventriculostomy catheter placement on a CT patient dataset using ImmersiveTouch with that of a recent retrospective evaluation study done at University of Missouri Hospital performed on the head CT scans of 97 patients who underwent 98 free-hand pass ventriculostomy

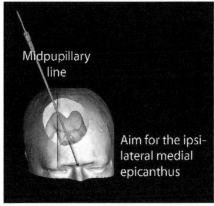
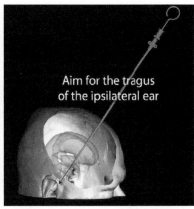

Landmark in the frontal plane **Landmark in the saggital plane**

Fig. 4. High-fidelity virtual reality and haptic procedures enabled by ImmersiveTouch high-fidelity simulator. (*Courtesy of* ImmersiveTouch, Chicago, IL.)

placements in an ICU setting. The average distance of the catheter tip to the foramen of Monro and the standard deviation were almost identical.

References

[1] Burt DE. Virtual reality in anaesthesia. Br J Anaesth 1995;75(4):472–80.
[2] Blezek DJ, Robb RA, Martin DP. Virtual reality simulation of regional anesthesia for training of residents. In: Proceedings of IEEE 33rd Hawaii International Conference on System Sciences; 2000.
[3] Hiemenz L, Stredney D, Schmalbrock P. Development of the force-feedback model for an epidural needle insertion simulator. Stud Health Technol Inform 1998;50:272–7.
[4] Stredney D, Sessanna D, McDonald JS, et al. A virtual simulation environment for learning epidural anesthesia. Stud Health Technol Inform 1996;29:164–75.
[5] SensAble technologies. Available at: http://www.sensable.com. Accessed February 2007.
[6] Eason MP. Simulation devices in cardiothoracic and vascular anesthesia. Semin Cardiothorac Vasc Anesth 2005;9(4):309–23.
[7] Rowe R, Cohen RA. An evaluation of a virtual reality airway simulator. Anesth Analg 2002; 95(1):62–6.
[8] Goldmann K, Steinfeldt T. Acquisition of basic fiberoptic intubation skills with a virtual reality airway simulator. J Clin Anesth 2006;18(3):173–8.
[9] Satava RM. Virtual reality for medical applications. In: Information technology applications in biomedicine, 1997. ITAB'97. Proceedings of the IEEE Engineering in Medicine and Biology Society Region 8 International Conference 1997:19–20.
[10] Gaba DM. Simulation-based crisis resource management training for trauma care. Am J Anesthesiol 2000;27:199–200.
[11] Accreditation Council for Graduate Medical Education (ACGME) Bulletin. December 2005.
[12] Banerjee P, Charbel F. On-demand high fidelity neurosurgical procedure simulator prototype at University of Illinois using virtual reality and haptics. ACGME Bulletin 2006; 20–1.

[13] Cruz-Neira C, Sandin DJ, DeFanti TA, et al. The CAVE: audio visual experience automatic virtual environment. Commun ACM 1992;35(6):65–72.

[14] Iowa State University. The most realistic virtual reality room in the world. Available at: http://www.iastate.edu/~nscentral/news/2006/may/c6update.shtml. Accessed February 2007.

[15] Czernuszenko M, Pape D, Sandin D, et al. The ImmersaDesk and infinity wall projection-based virtual reality displays. Comput Graph 1997.

[16] Planar systems, SD stereo/3D monitors. Available at: http://www.planar.com/products/flatpanel_monitors/stereoscopic/. Accessed February 2007.

[17] Johnson A, Sandin D, Dawe G, et al. Developing the PARIS: using the CAVE to prototype a new VR display. In: Proceedings of IPT 2000: Immersive Projection Technology Workshop, Ames (IA). 2000.

[18] Leigh J, Luciano C, Dawe G, et al. University of Illinois at Chicago, 2005. ImmersaDesk4 design. Available at: http://www.evl.uic.edu/cavern/rg/20050415_leigh. Accessed May 2007.

[19] Banerjee P, Luciano C, Florea L, et al. Compact haptic and augmented virtual reality device. U.S. Provisional Patent Application No. 60/646,837, March 2005. U.S. Patent Application, January 2006.

[20] Luciano C, Banerjee P, Florea L, et-al. Design of the ImmersiveTouch: a high-performance haptic augmented virtual reality system. In: Proc. of Human-Computer Interaction (HCI) International Conf. Las Vegas (NV): 2005.

[21] Luciano C, Banerjee P, Lemole GM Jr, et al. Second generation haptic ventriculostomy simulator using the ImmersiveTouch system. Stud Health Technol Inform 2006;119:343–8.

ELSEVIER
SAUNDERS

Anesthesiology Clin
25 (2007) 349–359

ANESTHESIOLOGY
CLINICS

Procedural Simulation

Aalpen A. Patel, MD[a],*, Craig Glaiberman, MD[b],
Derek A. Gould, MBChB, FRCP, FRCR[c]

[a]Department of Radiology, University of Pennsylvania School of Medicine,
Hospital of the University of Pennsylvania, One Silverstein,
3400 Spruce Street, Philadelphia, PA 19104, USA
[b]Mallinckrodt Institute of Radiology, Washington University School of Medicine,
510 South Kingshighway Boulevard, St Louis, MO 63110, USA
[c]Royal Liverpool University Hospital, Prescot Street, Liverpool L7 8XP, United Kingdom

The aviation industry realized the potential of simulation for training many decades ago and has harnessed its potential. In the past few decades, medicine has started to look at the potential use of simulators in medical education. Procedural medicine lends itself well to the use of simulators. This effort was put into high gear after 1999 when the Institute of Medicine Publication "To Err is Human: Building a Safer Healthcare System" [1] quantified medical errors and their consequences. It stated that up to 98,000 patients die each year because of medical errors in the United States alone. This led to heightened interest from governmental agencies, lay public, and doctors themselves. Efforts are under way to establish national agendas to change the way medical education is approached and thereby improve patient safety. Universities, credentialing organizations [2], and hospitals are investing large sums of money to build and use simulation centers for undergraduate and graduate medical education [2–4].

The aspiring trainee must somehow acquire the essential knowledge, core cognitive and motor skills, and professionalism that are required for safe practice in patients. The basic procedural skills are acquired through deliberate practice until they become automated; they can then be reconfigured and merged with new cognitive and motor elements to build up tasks that are more complex. This stepwise training is conducted within a curriculum

---

Procedural simulation should not be viewed independent of the other important topics in this issue. Understanding different types of simulators, their uses, links between simulation, and patient safety puts this important topic in perspective. This article may touch on these topics, but for detailed information please refer to other articles in this issue.

* Corresponding author.
E-mail address: aalpen.patel@uphs.upenn.edu (A.A. Patel).

where the master-apprentice model (MAM) has traditionally been a corner-stone. The mentor provides instruction, example, supervision, assessment, and safety through rescue-intervention. In the current system of medical education, it is rarely possible to master a skill through repeated practice of basic skills before "practicing" on patients [5]. The inexperienced trainee also needs to rely on these basic skills to perform complex procedures in a team environment. The safety of patients and procedural team members, and perhaps the outcome of the procedure, depends on a coordinated effort among team members and the chain of tasks they perform. Any disruption in the fluidity of these tasks may result in injury to a patient or team member with potentially grave consequences. Many experts believe that the MAM of medical education, where "see one, do one, teach one" is the mantra, is no longer a safe option and that medical education syllabi should incorporate the use of simulators to provide optimal patient safety. Despite its time-proved strengths, MAM has its weaknesses, leading some to conclude that it is time for a paradigm shift. For example, different trainees require different amounts of time to master a given skill. Furthermore, training varies depending on the case mix available at a particular training site [3,6].

Many instructors in medicine are not trained to be evaluators, and this may limit the reproducibility, reliability, and objectivity of their assessment of the trainee's proficiency. Further, a mainstay of training is learning from error, and it is indeed unfortunate that patients are at times subjected to the mistakes of trainees learning under supervision [3,4]. These shortcomings lead in turn to legal and ethical concerns, and pressure is mounting for a gradual change in medical education. Procedural medicine (interventional or surgical) education lends itself to change. Intuitively, it is a matter of risk/benefit ratio: the higher the risk of the procedure for the patient, the more benefit the patient obtains if he or she is not the tool for teaching. In addi-tion, procedural medicine carries inherent risk to the operating team mem-bers. Seymour and colleagues demonstrated that practice on an appropriate simulator leads to reduced errors in patients [7], and in the future, it may even be shown to improve patient outcomes and safety for team members. Simulators have a key role, not only in basic skills and individual training, but also in performing assessments of proficiency [3].

From this, one has an intuitive understanding of what medical simulation might represent and provide. The definitions differ with different investiga-tors and perspectives; however, there are some common threads. One defi-nition is creation of an environment or a group of environments in which cognitive and physical skills are acquired through the use of audiovisual media, devices, mannequins, or a team (or any combination of these) with or without the presence of a standardized patient. A simulator is a device, method, or audiovisual (or any combination of these) effect that allows all or part of the simulation to occur. With the currently available technology, the replacement of MAM is unlikely. Using a range of simulation methods, however, its augmentation is certainly possible. This augmentation should allow the trainee's early learning curve to be accelerated, allowing them to learn from errors on virtual, rather than real, patients. Incorporation of simulation in procedural medicine curriculum introduces a more moldable and adaptable element into the relatively rigid MAM, allowing it to meet specific performance objectives required for curricular training, objectively measuring indicators of performance to provide reliable and reproducible feedback on proficiency [3,4].

Procedural simulation: its potential and pitfalls

It is unquestioned that, if done in a responsible and careful manner, procedural simulation holds tremendous promise for the future of medical training. It must be recognized, however, that if not used properly, it has pitfalls.

Potential roles of procedural simulation

The potential uses of simulation in medicine, especially procedural medicine, are huge. With the simulators that are currently available, the replacement of MAM is unlikely in the near future. Some of the technologic issues (and fantastic potential) with this are reviewed by Banerjee and colleagues elsewhere in this issue in their description of futuristic virtual reality simulation techniques that are undergoing development. As technology is developed and subjected to validation, there will be gradual incorporation into educational curricula. Procedural simulators may be used for (1) aptitude testing; (2) teaching basic skills before patient interaction; (3) teaching advanced skills before performing complex procedures on patients; (4) procedure rehearsal on real patient anatomy loaded onto the simulator; (5) invention of new procedures (answering "what if I tried this?"); and (6) if done with an evidence basis, credentialing and certification. This is by no means a comprehensive list, but a taste of the possible roles. Almost every branch of procedural medicine, ranging from interventional radiology and vascular surgery, to gastrointestinal medicine, to orthopedic surgery, is exploring simulation for their unique uses [3,4].

Procedural simulations lie on a continuum ranging from part task physical model (low fidelity and passive) simulators to virtual reality or augmented reality simulators (high fidelity and active). In the near-term, because of financial and computational cost considerations, low-fidelity simulators may be useful to teach basic skills, reserving high-fidelity simulators to obtain the more intricate combinations of visual and tactile cues and cognitive and motor skills required to perform complex tasks [5]. The patient's own imaging data may be imported to high-fidelity procedural simulators. This allows "mission rehearsal" of difficult cases in a simulated environment before ever touching the patient. In these ways, simulation may bring great flexibility and safety in training, thereby becoming an indispensable tool in attaining, assessing, and maintaining higher levels of expertise than is currently possible in the traditional MAM [3,4,8].

Given the range of alternatives to practicing on patients that are becoming available, their requirements for relevant content and appropriate fidelity, and the ultimate need for validity to be demonstrable, it can be difficult to ascertain where and how they should be integrated into training. Patient and team safety must be the primary objectives, achieved by eliminating the early learning curve before the first attempt on patients. Although simulation seems to have an obvious role here, when considering a given simulator model for training, it is essential first to determine the development methodology used, and the curriculum on which the simulation is based. Even better, and to avoid unnecessary technology development, the curricular training objectives that actually require simulation should first be identified by subject experts. Once it is determined where simulation should fit with the curriculum, it is possible to determine which of these identified training objectives might be met by existing simulators, and even to effect focused simulator development, specific to the curriculum's requirements. The roles required of simulation should be determined at the design stage of a curriculum, and ideally this information used as a basis for simulator model design. It stands to reason that ultimately, minimum standards will be required in simulator use [3].

Credentialing

Time honored use of written and oral examinations lacks validity for assessing technical skills. High-stakes training requires reliable skills assessment, both for the security and safety of patients and the protection of the trainee. Computer-based simulation can provide a facility to record and evaluate an operator's performance automatically and reproducibly, removing the subjectivity and bias of assessments used in the current MAM. This performance feedback can help the operator develop and theoretically be evidence (summative) for a certification [9]. For simulation effectively to contribute to training and assessment in this way requires that the content of the simulation follows the discipline's curriculum [10], and that the assessment process meets requirements for reproducibility, cost effectiveness, and feasibility [11]. Potentially objective methods, such as checklists, global scoring systems, and standardized patients, have been used to assess proficiency in procedural medicine (surgery); the assessment of many other fields is frequently based on logbook record to show acquisition of experience and, it is hoped, skills [12–18]. This or any other subjective method does not always demonstrate proficiency and does not take into account the differing rates of learning. They are subject to the differing case mix and expertise among training sites. The previously described deficiencies may be addressed with the use of simulation with automated assessment of specific metrics of performance [7,19–21]. Procedural simulation has been used successfully in some surgical procedures (eg, laparoscopy).

Some assessments provided in current simulators use general measures of overall performance, such as time to completion. While such "high level" metrics may infer some indication of skill, measures of detailed actions and errors relevant to specific performance objectives are often lacking. This may be the result of several factors including possible lack of robust input from a group of subject matter experts, or the inability to implement or use additional metrics by the current state of a particular simulator's technology. Detailed and more relevant metrics are yet to be clearly identified for many procedural fields, however, and this requires knowledge of what is happening in the real world task. This can be based on careful collection of video records of procedures performed by recognized subject matter experts. A psychologist is then engaged to detail the skills used, and then, in a further interview of subject experts, to identify the cues, decisions, and psychomotor actions, which comprise the task that was originally performed. This Physical and Cognitive Task Analysis forms the basis of an analysis to identify which procedure steps are most critical and most prone to error: these data can be used as metrics to evaluate the learner's proficiency [3,22–25].

Potential pitfalls

Having proved itself in aviation, space exploration, and industrial applications, simulation is poised to become an important augment to training and assessment in procedural medicine. While adopting it, the educators must keep in mind the potential pitfalls so they can be avoided during development and implementation. Inadvertently overstating or aggressively interpreting the evidence is a pitfall that must be avoided. Whenever possible, the evidence must be collected in a rigorous fashion. The evidence may be obtained by the "use, validate, improve" model. That is, one begins to use these devices along with traditional training, obtain validation evidence while using it, and improve the simulator or curricula if needed. One must also consider some ethical issues. The question is, validate or not to validate. Is anything other than full-fledged implementation, without evidence specific to the simulators in use, unethical? Does transitivity apply in a setting of proved use of simulation in other fields? Will the attempt to obtain the "holy grail" (ie, transfer of training) obtained with a randomized study put patients at an additional risk? These are not easy questions, nor are they free of controversy, but they must be addressed.

Another important question is, if not used carefully, does the use of simulation for training potentially thwart or limit creativity? The different but safe ways of performing procedures, by different operators, must be taken into account when defining metrics and designing curriculum for procedural simulation. Involving subject matter experts from different specialties helps address this issue and creates a more robust set of metrics. Will an improperly designed curriculum teach the trainee bad habits? For example, if "short cuts" are permitted and used during the training on the simulator, the trainee may inadvertently use these same short cuts on patients, placing the patient and team at risk, defeating the goal of the procedural simulation [3,4].

Another potential pitfall is the difficulty providing adequate and meaningful feedback to trainees, which a simulator currently cannot do. This requires a large amount of time and dedication on the part of academic physicians with already busy clinical schedules. Finding the means to insert additional curricula into overtaxed residency requirements is difficult. This is particularly paramount in the face of current "duty hour" restrictions. One option may be to lengthen training programs such that they can include dedicated time for simulation.

One must also consider potential pitfalls that are not always thought of. Since the advent of virtual reality, simulator sickness has been recognized. Although the definition is controversial, symptoms range from nausea and dizziness to sleepiness and apathy [26,27]. It is a well known phenomenon in head-mounted displays [28], but does this exist in procedural simulation?

Simulator design considerations

As a larger point of view, several factors must be considered in design of simulators. It is imperative that the purpose of a procedural simulator is defined in detail, including task requirements; metrics requirement; software environment; hardware and interface (GUI, haptics, and physical interface); and specifications. There may be multiple valid pathways or sequences of steps to perform a procedure, making the definition of a task or procedure difficult. This should also be considered when identifying metrics so that trainees are not penalized for constructive imagination. Task analysis performed with an educational psychologist is crucial in obtaining this information. This information gathering must also be dynamic and evolve with improved procedural techniques and tool change [3,29].

Many validation studies can be performed to determine how relevant the simulation is to performance of the real world procedure or task. For training purposes content validity ("accurate replication of the procedure it claims to model") and face validity ("appearing to test takers to resemble the real world task") [3] is important. To attain face and content validity, the simulation must clearly provide an appropriate level of fidelity. For assessment purposes, however, benchmarks and construct validity are more important. This allows the simulator properly to distinguish the performance of experts from that of novices. It is not enough, however, to demonstrate that performance improves on a simulator. The assessment should be able to predict future performance and competence (predictive validation), confirmed by a separate clinical study. For integration into curricula, face and content validity are particularly important, but the use of simulation for assessment requires at least face, construct, and content validity. Once this has been shown, it seems more likely that skills developed in the simulation will transfer to the conditions of real world procedures in patients, and be maintained over time. This specific benchmark is known as "transfer of training" (or skills transfer).

Although there exist claims of successful validation, few simulators have yet to show improvement in technical skills in patients [29–32]. Virtual reality to operating room evidence exists for laparoscopic simulation [7], for example, but is noticeably lacking in endovascular simulators [29]. It is only a matter of time when further development and validation of simulators will effectively augment the deficiencies in MAM, reducing the use of patients as practice subjects.

Standards

The recent drive to develop and incorporate medical simulation in education has been caused by patient safety concerns. Because of this, the simulation industry has begun to assume a duly deserved center stage in the medical education arena. Because they have limited financial resources, there may be collaborative opportunities for academia and governmental agencies in the development and validation of simulators. The educational institutions must take the lead and set standards for validation, standards for procedural simulation use in their curricula, and even broader device development standards.

Standards for curriculum

There is a fundamental need to now unravel the nature of skills, and the level of fidelity required for their acquisition. It is inescapable that for any practitioner, surgeon, radiologist, or cardiologist to learn relevant skills that transfer to real world tasks in patients, the training environment must have an appropriate level of sensory fidelity, content that mirrors the real world task, and evidence-based metrics that test technical skills. Thus equipped, computer-based simulation should train and assess actual skills required, without the risk of training inappropriate or incorrect skills (negative training) and with greater likelihood of successful, clinical validation.

Based on this, there may be a need to redefine training curricula to identify insertion sites for simulation that meet specific training objectives. A number of the radiological societies have formed individual simulation taskforces and a combined Joint International Task Force to outline a strategy for using simulation methodologies to help train and assess interventional radiologists. Similar efforts are already underway in other specialties. However, such efforts need to occur not only in specialties in isolation, but also collaboratively, across specialties. The difficulties in achieving this include attaining consensus, professional competition, and other political issues. Yet, uniform curriculum standards for specialties performing identical or similar procedures would bring great logistical benefits for creators of simulations of these interventions.

Simulator development standards

A unified standard that facilitates upgrades and allows communication between different simulators is essential for advancement of simulator technology. Cross-platform communication and compatibility may prove to be invaluable for team training using simulation. For example, when performing a procedure under anesthesia, simulated by an appropriate anesthesia simulator, it would be helpful if the procedural simulator were able to communicate with the anesthesia simulator. These may be made by different companies but compliance with appropriate standards would allow the communication. If a complication occurred during the procedural simulation, the anesthesia simulator would detect the change in the patient's physiology and the anesthesiologist would react appropriately. Those involved in simulation, including academicians and educators, industry partners, and end users, have started to assess the future need for a unified, open software, hardware, and interface standards. On the software side, at least two such efforts are underway. First is Simulation Open Framework Architecture, with a goal to create an open software platform for medical simulator development [33]. Second is an effort by the Scientific Computing and Imaging Institute of the University of Utah, the Unified Virtual Environment. It would be ideal to unify such efforts for standardization and advancement of simulator efforts [3].

Similarly, a hardware development framework and standard architecture, defining computational platform and human-computer interface, are needed. An interface analogous to "plug and play with USB on personal computers" is also critical. These types of efforts may help prevent duplication of resources. Such standardization may help foster smaller companies that lack the resources of larger companies yet are placed to develop niche simulators to fill needs not yet addressed by their larger counterparts. It may also help drive competition and innovation [3].

Using simulators within a curriculum

It is axiomatic that knowledge of the subject, cognitive and technical skills, and judgment skills are prerequisites in successful procedural medicine practice. Each simulator in theory should be validated, although given rapidly changing technology, limited funding, and time, it may not be possible or practical to validate all simulated tasks to demonstrate transfer of skills. The authors propose that, although it may not be possible to validate all, one can increase the probability of a valid simulator by designing them properly. The "transfer of training" is more likely to be demonstrable if the simulator had appropriate fidelity, valid content, and metrics. Although predictive validation remains an important yardstick, uptake of properly developed simulations will lead to circumstances that favor validation, and in turn validation will drive increased use. Therefore, if such simulations are used cautiously as a supplement to, rather than a replacement of, the MAM, validation should become more attainable, with a return on this investment of enhanced patient safety.

Although cautiously using the simulator, curriculum should not be neglected. The curriculum provides a variety of training and assessment tools, providing checks and balances. Use of simulation without curriculum is meaningless. The broad curriculum provides "reliable scope of training and ultimate sanction of certification: simulation would, at least for the foreseeable future, form but a part of this 'big picture'" [3]. Until the technology advances conceivably to provide automated mentorship, it is the human mentor that provides an assessment, with simulation introducing objectivity. Simulation should not be used as a stand-alone training methodology.

The horizon and beyond

The incorporation of procedural simulation in medical education curriculum, in one form or another, is inevitable. The strategies for its incorporation and implementation depend on many factors, and these factors influence the time to maturity. Funding is the most important factor in these endeavors. The spirit of research, willingness of investigators to collaborate, and the willingness of governmental agencies to recognize the limitations of the current medical educational system, however, dictate how long it takes to exploit procedural simulation's full potential. In the future, scenarios will range from using the procedural tools themselves, to gathering metrics, to evaluating performance while working on real patients, to completely immersive simulation (akin to Star Trek's "Holodeck") [3].

The American Board of Surgery has already mandated incorporation of simulation in its curriculum starting in 2008 [34]. The American Society of Anesthesiologists has convened a 21-member Workgroup on Simulation Education, which has produced a comprehensive white paper on simulation in anesthesiology [35,36]. In addition, this committee has recommended the formation of a standing committee of the American Society of Anesthesiologists. Simulation has not penetrated the curriculum requirements by the American Board of Anesthesiology or by the Anesthesiology residency review committee of the Accreditation Council of Graduate Medical Education. Others, such as the Joint International Taskforce of the Society of Interventional Radiology, and the Cardiovascular and Interventional Society of Europe, have already written a strategy for simulation, and are working on implementation [37]. Funding, however, remains an issue in this relative infancy of simulation. Governmental agencies need to step up and fund the effort to develop, validate, and introduce simulation into medical education. It is the moral responsibility of the educators, hospitals, and overseeing governmental agencies to develop and implement simulation strategies for the safety of the patient and the operating team, and perhaps better education for the trainee.

References

[1] Kohn JT, Corrigan JM, Donaldson MS. To err is human: building a safer healthcare system. Washington, DC: National Academy Press; 1999.
[2] Royal College of Radiologists integrated training initiative. Available at: http://www.riti. org.uk/. Accessed May 3, 2007.
[3] Patel AA, Gould DA. Simulators in interventional radiology training and evaluation: a paradigm shift is on the horizon. J Vasc Interv Radiol 2006;17:S163–73.
[4] Dawson S. Procedural simulation: a primer. J Vasc Interv Radiol 2006;17:205–13.
[5] Dankelman J, Chmarra MK, Verdaasdonk EGG, et al. Fundamental aspects of learning minimally invasive surgical skills–review. Minim Invasive Ther Allied Technol 2005; 14(4/5):247–56.
[6] Villegas L, Schneider BE, Callery MP, et al. Laparoscopic skills training. Surg Endosc 2003; 17:1879–88.
[7] Seymour NE, Gallagher AG, Roman SA, et al. Virtual reality training improves operating room performance: results of a randomized, double-blinded study. Ann Surg 2002;236(4): 458–63 [discussion 463–4].
[8] Cates CU, Patel AD, Nicholson WJ. Use of virtual reality simulation for mission rehearsal for carotid stenting. JAMA 2007;297(3):265–6.
[9] Southgate L, Grant J. Principles for an assessment system for postgraduate medical training. A working paper for the Postgraduate Medical Education Training Board. September 2004.
[10] Dauphinee WD. Licensure and certification. In: Norman GR, Van der Vleuten CPM, Newlble DI, editors. International handbook of research in medical education, Part 2. Dordrecht (The Netherlands): Kluwer Academic Publishers; 2002. p. 836.
[11] Shumway JM, Harden RM. AMEE Guide No. 25: the assessment of learning outcomes for the competent and reflective physician. Medical Teacher 2003;25(6):569–84.
[12] Kneebone R, Kidd J, Nestel D, et al. Blurring the boundaries: scenario-based simulation in a clinical setting. Med Educ 2005;39:580–7.
[13] Datta V, Bann S, Beard J, et al. Comparison of bench test evaluations of surgical skill with live operating performance assessments. J Am Coll Surg 2004;199(4):603–6.
[14] Faulkner H, Regehr G, Martin J, et al. Validation of an objective structured assessment of technical skill for surgical residents. Acad Med 1996;71:1363–5.
[15] Moorthy K, Munz Y, Sarker SK, et al. Objective assessment of technical skills in surgery. BMJ 2003;327:1032–7.
[16] Cushieri A, Francis N, Crosby J, et al. What do master surgeons think of surgical competence and revalidation? Am J Surg 2001;182:110–6.
[17] European Association of Endoscopic Surgeons: training and assessment of competence. Surg Endosc 1994;8:721–2.
[18] Battles JB, Wilkinson SL, Lee SJ. Using standardized patients in an objective structured clinical examination as a patient safety tool. Qual Saf Health Care 2004;13(Suppl 1):i46–50.
[19] Taffinder N, Sutton C, Fishwick RJ, et al. Validation of virtual reality to teach and assess psychomotor skills in laparoscopic surgery: results from randomised controlled studies using the MIST VR laparoscopic simulator. Studies in Health Technology & Informatics 1998;50: 124–30.
[20] Gallagher AG, Cates CU. Virtual reality training for the operating room and cardiac catheterisation laboratory. Lancet 2004;364:1538–40.

[21] Sherman KP, Ward JW, Wills DP, et al. Surgical trainee assessment using a VE knee arthroscopy training system (VE-KATS): experimental results. Studies in Health Technology & Informatics 2001;81:465–70.
[22] Clark RE, Estes F. Cognitive task analysis for training. Int J Educ Res 1996;25(5):403–17.
[23] Grunwald T, Clark D, Fisher SS, et al. Using cognitive task analysis to facilitate collaboration in development of simulators to accelerate surgical training. In: Westwood JD, Haluck RS, Hoffman HM, et al, editors. Medicine meets virtual reality 12. Amsterdam (The Netherlands): IOS Press; 2004. p. 114–20.
[24] Johnson SJ, Healey AE, Evans JC, et al. Physical and cognitive task analysis in interventional radiology. Clin Radiol 2006;61(1):97–103.
[25] Lewandowski W. Performing a task analysis–the critical step in creating a simulation that improves human performance. In: Proceedings Medicine Meets Virtual Reality 12 Conference, Newport Beach (CA); 2004.
[26] Ebenholtz SM. Motion sickness and oculomotor systems in virtual environments. Presence 1992;1:302–5.
[27] Pausch R, Crea T, Conway M. A literature survey for virtual environments: military flight simulator visual systems and simulator sickness. Presence 1992;1:344–63.
[28] DiZio P, Lackner JR. Spatial orientation, adaptation, and motion sickness in real and virtual environments. Presence 1992;1:319–28.
[29] Gould DA, Kessel DO, Healey AE, et al. Simulators in catheter based interventional radiology: training or computer games? Clin Radiol 2006;61:556–61.
[30] Hsu JH, Younan D, Pandalai S, et al. Use of computer simulation for determining endovascular skill levels in a carotid stenting model. J Vasc Surg 2004;40(6):1118–24.
[31] Dayal R, Faries PL, Lin SC, et al. Computer simulation as a component of catheter based training. J Vasc Surg 2004;40(6):1112–7.
[32] Agarwal R, Black SA, Hance JR, et al. Virtual reality simulation can improve inexperienced surgeon's endovascular skills. Eur J Endovasc Surg 2006;31:588–93.
[33] Simulation open framework architecture. Available at: http://sofa-framework.org. Accessed July 16, 2006.
[34] Education and training committee to develop National curriculum ABS news. 2004. Available at: http://home.absurgery.org/xfer/newslet2004winter.pdf. Accessed February 21, 2007.
[35] ASA approval of simulation programs. ASA workgroup on simulation education. 2006. Available at: http://www.asahq.org/ASASimWhitePaper031506.pdf. Accessed February 21, 2007.
[36] Workgroup on Simulation Education (COE). Report to the house of delegates of the American Society of Anesthesiologists. 2006. Available at: http://www.asahq.org/SIM/SIMReporttoHOD8-29-06.pdf. Accessed February 21, 2007.
[37] SIR and CIRSE joint medical simulation task force strategic plan. Available at: http://www.cirse.org/_files/contentmanagement/CIRSE_SIR_Joint_Strategy.pdf. Accessed February 21, 2007.

ANESTHESIOLOGY
CLINICS

Anesthesiology Clin
25 (2007) 361–376

Debriefing with Good Judgment: Combining Rigorous Feedback with Genuine Inquiry

Jenny W. Rudolph, PhD[a,c,*], Robert Simon, EdD[c,d,e],
Peter Rivard, PhD[b], Ronald L. Dufresne, PhD[f],
Daniel B. Raemer, PhD[c,d,e]

[a]*Department of Health Policy and Management, Boston University School of Public Health,
715 Albany Street, Boston, MA 02118–2526, USA*
[b]*Center for Organization, Leadership and Management Research, VA Boston Healthcare
System, 150 South Huntington Avenue (152M), Boston, MA 02130, USA*
[c]*Center for Medical Simulation, 65 Landsdowne Street, Cambridge, MA 02139, USA*
[d]*Harvard Medical School, 25 Shattuck Street, Boston, MA 02115, USA*
[e]*Massachusetts General Hospital, Department of Anesthesia and Critical Care,
55 Fruit Street, Boston, MA 02114, USA*
[f]*Department of Management, Haub School of Business, St. Joseph's University,
5600 City Avenue, Philadelphia, PA 19131, USA*

Reflection on one's own practice is a crucial step in the experiential learning process. It helps trainees develop and integrate insights from direct experience into later action [1,2]. Subsequent to participating in a simulated case, debriefing or after-action review provides a way for clinicians using medical simulation to do this reflection. There is convergence in the debriefing literature on some of the important goals and processes of such debriefing. The goals are to allow trainees to explain, analyze, and synthesize information and emotional states to improve performance in similar situations in the future. The process for achieving these goals usually follows a series of steps, such as processing reactions, analyzing the situation, generalizing to everyday experience, and shaping future action by lessons learned [3–11].

How to create a debriefing environment in which trainees feel both challenged and psychologically safe enough [12] to engage in rigorous reflection

---

* Corresponding author. Department of Health Policy and Management, Boston University School of Public Health, 715 Albany Street, Boston, MA 02118–2526.
E-mail address: jrudolph@bu.edu (J.W. Rudolph).

1932-2275/07/$ - see front matter © 2007 Elsevier Inc. All rights reserved.
doi:10.1016/j.anclin.2007.03.007   *anesthesiology.theclinics.com*

is generally left unspecified. Sharing critical judgments is an essential part of learning in simulation and debriefing. Yet, instructors often avoid giving voice to critical thoughts and feelings because they do not want to seem confrontational and they worry that criticism might lead to hurt feelings or defensiveness on the part of the trainee. Voicing critical judgment poses a dilemma for many instructors (eg, "How can I deliver a critical message and share my expertise while avoiding negative emotions, preserving social face and maintaining my relationship with the trainee?"). This article offers an approach to debriefing that addresses this dilemma.

By "rigorous reflection" we mean a debriefing process that brings to the surface and helps resolve the clinical and behavioral dilemmas and areas of confusion raised by the simulation experience. Drawing on a 35-year research program on improving professional effectiveness in the business world through "reflective practice" [11–17], this article articulates a model of debriefing for medical simulation exercises. The research program from which the approach is adapted has studied and helped thousands of practicing business executives and managers improve their personal and interpersonal effectiveness through the discipline of reflective practice.[1] The debriefing model adapted from this work has three primary components. The first component is a conceptual framework, drawn from research in cognitive science and on reflective practice, that guides the instructor on how to illuminate the mental models that were salient in guiding trainees' actions during the simulation. The second is an underlying debriefing stance that unites the apparently contradictory values of curiosity about and respect for the trainee and the value of clear evaluative judgments about trainee performance. The third component is a way of talking (combining advocacy and inquiry) that enacts the underlying stance.

The basis of this article is the literature in the field of reflective practice and the authors' experience with exercising the debriefing with good judgment approach. All of the authors use this approach regularly and four have together conducted approximately 2000 debriefings using this method. Over the last 2 years they have trained nearly 300 medical educators to use this approach. Most medical educators are able reliably to demonstrate competence after approximately 2 days of lecture and practice; expertise seems to require considerably longer to develop. Of the approximately 20 teaching faculty who regularly use simulation as an educational technique at the authors' simulation center, approximately half use the debriefing with good judgment approach. The other half has not yet been trained in its use. Faculty who are comfortable with the technique find their skills quite stable and robust in the face of a great variety of trainees.

---

[1] "Reflective practice" is a term coined by the late MIT professor Donald Schön, to describe the discipline of examining the values, assumptions, and knowledge-base that drives one's own professional practice [11,12,19,20].

Reflective practice: method and theory

Reflective practice is a method used to scrutinize one's own professional work practices and the taken-for-granted assumptions that underlie them. It is often accomplished in a collaborative setting [16]: in this case, the relevant setting is the simulation debriefing wherein colleagues and trainees are helped to develop crisis resource management, clinical, and reflective practice skills. Researchers at Harvard University and the Massachusetts Institute of Technology developed the method as part of their investigation of how to support students in their professional schools and also to help experienced professionals to develop self-correcting versus self-sealing practice habits [18]. They found that reflective practitioners, who learned to scrutinize their taken-for-granted assumptions and mental routines, were able to self-correct and improve their professional skills. Those without skill in this self-scrutiny, however, tended to seal out or ignore disconfirming data and maintained ineffective habits of practice [11,12,14,19,20].

The theory underlying reflective practice draws on cognitive science, social psychology, and anthropology. The central idea is that people make sense of external stimuli through internal cognitive frames, internal images of external reality [20–25]. Terms for these images are myriad: "frames of reference," "schemata," and "mental models," to name a few. People do not passively perceive an objective reality, but engage in sensemaking by which they actively filter, create, and apply meaning to their environment [26–28]. For example, a diagnosis becomes a frame for subsequent actions, as do assumptions, such as, "It's not a good idea to discuss mistakes here, or "I must have a bag-mask apparatus to ventilate this patient." Fig. 1 shows the relationships among frames, actions, and simulation results.

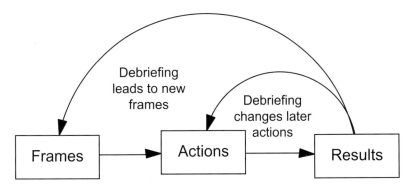

Fig. 1. Frames are invisible, but inferable; they are in the mind of trainees and of instructors. Actions (including speech) are observable. Most results (eg, vital signs, order or chaos) are also observable.

These frames, in turn, shape the actions people take. Both clinical frames and social or interpersonal frames can play crucial roles in medical decision making. A trauma physician facing a patient with a ventilation problem, for example, takes one set of actions if they frame the symptoms as a physical obstruction of the airway and another if their diagnosis is reactive airway disease. A nurse who holds the frame that reporting an error leads to punishment reports errors at a very different rate than one who believes the report is used to improve work processes [29]. Or, in an example used throughout this article, consider an anesthesiologist who is called to manage an unresponsive patient in a setting where a bag-mask apparatus is not readily available. They hold the frame that they can only resuscitate using the device with which they are most familiar, a bag mask, and delay treatment while the patient descends into hypoxemia and arrest. The model suggests that people's actions, including those of this anesthesiologist, are an inevitable result of how they frame the situation they face.

Importantly, even mistakes are usually the result of intentionally rational actions [23,27,30]. That is, the actions make perfect sense given how the person was framing the situation at that moment. Continuing the example of the anesthesiologist, the instructor may be surprised that instead of considering passive oxygenation or delivering a mouth-to-mask "rescue breath," the anesthesiologist trainee searched relentlessly for a bag-mask apparatus while the patient desaturated. These actions make perfect sense, however, when the instructor understands that the trainee held the belief that basic life support cannot be achieved without a bag-mask device, mouth-to-mouth was out of the question, and passive oxygenation is something that he has never learned. It is the instructor's job during a debriefing to help the trainee bring these frames to the surface; analyze their impact on actions; and craft new frames (eg, if I do not find a bag-mask apparatus quickly, I have other options for ventilating) and actions (giving mouth-to-mask breaths, or apply oxygen and mechanically optimize the airway opening). In practice, the instructor asks questions during the debriefing to elicit these frames.

"Results," in the reflective practice model, are seen to be prompted by the actions the trainee takes. Results are states (eg, the patient's cardiac rhythm, whether the trainee ended up knowing the cause of the clinical problem, or whether there was chaos or order in the clinical environment). The instructor and the trainee usually have an implicit idea of what the desired results were. For example, the patient remains stable and does not go into cardiac arrest, the trainee and others know why the patient arrested in the first place, or the resuscitation ran smoothly. Learning occurs when instructor and trainee explore the frames-actions-results causal sequence in reverse. The instructor then explores with the trainee what frames and linked actions led to the actual results and then, as depicted in the feedback arrows in Fig. 1, collaborates with the trainee in developing alternative frames and actions for the future [16].

Debriefing stance: moving from judgmental debriefing to debriefing with good judgment

Although it may be obvious how discovering trainees' frames can enhance debriefing in medical simulation, the importance of identifying and revealing the instructor's frames is less obvious. Crucial to the process of a rigorous debriefing that is both nonthreatening and direct is instructors' learning to identify and examine their own frames related to the simulation they observed. Without an understanding of their own frames, instructors are handicapped in their ability to help illuminate a trainee's frames. The reasons for this are twofold. First, the instructors must be able to draw from their own experience the frames and actions they themselves might have deployed in a similar situation and to disclose these to the participant. Second, instructors have to be willing to test the validity of their own frames about the trainee's performance with trainees. To explain how this works, the authors start by describing and contrasting instructors' underlying frames when they are using judgmental, nonjudgmental, and debriefing with good judgment approaches (Table 1).

The judgmental approach to debriefing

Imagine or recall the instructor whose voice, dripping with disdain, inquires of a group of students, "Can anyone tell me what went wrong here?" or "Can anyone tell me Pat's big mistake?" The judgmental approach, whether laced with harsh criticism or more gently applied, places truth solely in the possession of the instructor, error in the hands of the trainee, and presumes that there is an essential failure in the thinking or actions of the trainee. In the last 15 years, the discourse in medical journals suggests that many clinicians concerned about reducing medical error and improving patient safety have sought to move health care away from the "shame and blame" approach captured in this style of questioning [31,32]. A judgmental approach to debriefing, especially one that includes harsh criticism, can have serious costs: humiliation, dampened motivation, reluctance to raise questions about later areas of confusion, or exit of talented trainees from the specialty or clinical practice altogether. But the shame and blame approach has an important virtue: the trainee is rarely left in doubt about what the instructor believes are the salient issues.

The nonjudgmental approach to debriefing

Some instructors shy away from a shame and blame approach to expressing their critical feelings and move toward a nonjudgmental approach. The central dilemma facing instructors who want to move away from this judgmental approach is how to deliver a critical message while avoiding negative emotions and defensiveness, preserving social face, and maintaining trust

Table 1
Contrasting judgmental, nonjudgmental, and good judgment approaches to debriefing

	Judgmental	Nonjudgmental	Debriefing with Good Judgment
The effective instructor	Gets the trainee to change	Gets the trainee to change	Creates a context for learning (and change)
Primary focus of debriefing	External: the actions or inactions of the other person	External: the actions or inactions of the other person	Internal: the meanings and assumptions of both instructor and trainee
How the trainee is seen	A mistake maker; a doer of actions	A mistake maker; a doer of actions	A meaning maker whose actions are the consequence of specific assumptions and knowledge
Who has the truth of the situation?	The instructor	The instructor	Possibly neither, either, or both
Who does not understand?	The trainee; "I (the instructor) will set you straight"	The trainee; "I (the instructor) will find the kindest way of filling you in on how to do this right."	The instructor: "I see what you are doing or not doing, and given my view, I don't get it"; or "Given my view, it seems problematic; what am I missing here?" Genuine report of puzzlement and inquiry into how the trainee's actions can make sense.

Basic stance toward self and trainee	"I'm right" or "You're wrong."	"I'm right" or "You're wrong" but, "I don't want you to get defensive so how do I tell you the bad news and get you to change in a nice way?"	Respect for self (I have a take on what happened in this simulation; that does lead me to think there were some problems but…)
	"I'm setting you straight"	"I'm setting you straight"	Respect for trainee (you are also a smart, well-trained practitioner, trying to do the right thing, who has your own view on the simulation) so…
	"I'm teaching you"	"I'm teaching you"	I am going to approach this as a genuine puzzle; not paralysis or indecision, but holding my own view tentatively. I seek clarity by honest inquiry (we both may learn something or change our minds); "Help me understand why you…?"
Typical message	"Here's how you messed up."	"What do you think you could have done better?"	"I noticed X. I was concerned about that because Y. I wonder how you saw it?"

Adapted from Kegan R, Lahey LL. How the way we talk can change the way we work. San Francisco (CA): Jossey-Bass; 2001. p. 134–5; with permission.

and psychological safety.[2] Instructors using a nonjudgmental approach often resolve the dilemma by using protective social strategies, such as the sandwich approach in which a compliment is followed by a criticism, which is, in turn, followed by another compliment; filtering out critical insights; or by avoiding the problem topic altogether [33,34]. Another common way for instructors to avoid the judgmental approach is to choose silence and express no critical thoughts or feelings. When people choose silence or nonjudgmental approaches that obscure their expert critique, important insights or feelings related to the trainee's performance remain murky or unexpressed. This deprives the trainee clinicians, and their organizations, of information that could improve how they work [35]. Avoiding critical thoughts and feelings also limits debriefings to safe-appearing, nonthreatening topics and leaves crucial areas of learning untouched [23].

Many instructors, ourselves included, have used a Socratic approach in which leading questions are asked and a kind tone of voice is used to guide the trainee to the critical insight the instructor holds but is reluctant to state explicitly. In his critique of this approach, Argyris [23] has termed it "easing in." The authors have found that when the instructor holds a critical judgment, open-ended or Socratic questions that camouflage the judgment may backfire. The trainee may become confused by the question or (justifiably) suspicious about the instructor's unexplained motives.

Although the nonjudgmental approach has the advantage of being nonblaming, and avoids some of the hurt and humiliation generated by the judgmental approach, it has serious weaknesses. Despite a desire to seem nonjudgmental, hints of one's views often leak by subtle cues, such as facial expression, tenor, cadence, and body language. Furthermore and most importantly, it is not nonjudgmental. Although the surface tone of nonjudgmental debriefing may be softer than the judgmental approach, as illustrated in Table 1, the underlying assumptions are the same: I'm right; I have the complete picture; my job is to hand off the correct knowledge or behavior to you, the trainee. Whereas the judgmental approach often humiliates directly, the nonjudgmental approach conveys nonverbally that mistakes are not discussable, or possibly shameful [36,37], undermining the very values (mistakes are puzzles to be learned from rather than crimes to be covered up) instructors aim to endorse with the nonjudgmental approach.

---

[2] Psychological safety is a person's sense that the immediate environment is safe for interpersonal risk taking; that trying out new ways of talking or acting will not be ridiculed; that mistakes will be worked on together as a source of learning instead of being treated as a crime to be punished or covered up [10,23].

Debriefing with good judgment approach

The debriefing with good judgment approach shifts the focus of debriefing in several ways.[3] First, it focuses on creating a psychologically safe context that enables adult learners (including the instructor) to move toward key learning objectives, determined either unilaterally by the instructor or collaboratively with the trainee. Second, the focus of the debriefing widens to include not only the trainee's actions, but also the meaning-making systems of the trainee (ie, their frames, assumptions, and knowledge). Third, the instructor's sense-making system about the simulation also becomes part of the debriefing terrain and open to question (see Table 1). The instructor has an expert's view of the situation that he or she shares to initiate dialog with the trainee, but it may not be the only valid view. Instructors' stating their main concerns in a debriefing is especially important in the domain of health care simulation where being indirect about crucial errors can perpetuate clinical mistakes and undermine patient safety when the trainee returns to the real clinical environment.[4] In this approach, in contrast to the nonjudgmental approach, the instructor shares critical or appreciative insights about the simulation explicitly. Then these insights are tested and explored with trainees step-by-step as illustrated in the next section and in Box 1. This "good judgment" approach is one that values the expert opinion of the instructors, while at the same time valuing the unique perspective of each trainee. The idea is to learn what frames drive trainee behaviors so that both their failures and successes can be understood as an ingenious, inevitable, and logical solution to the problem as perceived within their frames. This

---

[3] We offer a brief rationale of why we arrived at this framework. When our center started 12 years ago we relied on a nonjudgmental approach. To maintain a positive relationship with trainees, we thought it necessary to withhold judgment and use open-ended and leading questions in the hopes that the participants would arrive at the conclusions we were reluctant to say. We began to become uncomfortable with the approach when we realized that we were not "walking our talk." That is, we were saying that mistakes were discussable and a source of learning, yet we found that we tended to cover them up or shy away from discussing them. This conflicted with our commitment and stated mission to make errors discussable and enhance patient safety. We thought to ourselves, "If we can't discuss errors here in a simulation center, how can we expect others in the medical world to do it?" We believed that if we were going to advocate for patient safety, then we had to find a way to discuss errors openly; by the same token, we had to find a way respectfully to insert our clinical and behavioral expertise into our debriefings. We migrated to a position of "debriefing with good judgment," which allowed us, it seemed, the best of all worlds: it fit with educational theory; it allowed our participants to make mistakes and believe that they were still worthwhile and intelligent; it allowed us to use our clinical and behavioral expertise; and it fostered deep learning among our participants and instructors.

[4] In cases where the instructor has significant concerns about the trainee's clinical judgment or motives, concerns that might merit remedial training, counseling, or discipline, these are best treated in a follow-up. That is, if the instructor needs to convey that certain clinical approaches or social behaviors are not tolerated in the program, that message—a very important one—is a good topic for a postdebriefing conversation.

Box 1. Example of using advocacy-inquiry to elicit trainee's frames

Instructor says, "So, Damon, I noticed that you stepped away from the patient to find the bag-mask apparatus as the vital signs were deteriorating. I was thinking there possibly were alternative means to oxygenate the patient (advocacy). So I'm curious: how were you seeing the situation at that time? (inquiry)"

Damon replies,

"Actually yes, I knew what was going on, I had heard the saturation monitor decline earlier and I knew it was not going to get better on its own. I did not care what the actual reading was, which is why I figured I really needed ventilation equipment."

An instructor might then say, "Okay, that seems reasonable. I saw you looking all around the room for equipment, though, and that seemed to prevent you from trying any alternative approaches to oxygenating the patient (advocacy). Can you help me understand what you were considering at the time? (inquiry)"

When Damon replies, "Well, since breathing comes before circulation, I needed the manual resuscitator before doing anything else," the instructor is starting to surface the trainee's frame that he can only help a patient breathe if he has a bag-mask apparatus, and a valuable discussion point, linked specifically to the trainee's need, emerges. The instructor can now pursue such questions as: Does one always need a bag-mask apparatus to oxygenate a patient? What other options does one have? Will apneic oxygenation be sufficient in the short run? Will chest compressions provide adequate ventilation? What are the risks and benefits of mouth-to-mouth, mouth-to-mask, mouth-to-tube, or other rescue methods? If one is committed to manual ventilation, how does one manage personnel to get the proper equipment in the room expeditiously?

---

is where the instructor's stance is like that of an anthropologist, curious about different worldviews or frames and about the resulting actions.

Transparent talk in debriefing: enacting the good judgment approach with advocacy-inquiry

The debriefing with good judgment frames outlined in Table 1 are enacted by the style of speaking used by the instructor. Like all frames, mental models, or schemata, the values underlying the good judgment approach are invisible; the only way to see them is when they are transformed into

actions, and speaking is a powerful action for instructors. One particularly
effective style of debriefing speech is to pair advocacy with inquiry. An advocacy is an assertion, observation, or statement, whereas an inquiry is
a question. When pairing the two together, the instructor acts as a conversational scientist, stating in the advocacy his or her hypothesis, and then testing the hypothesis with an inquiry. For example, an instructor might say,
"So, Damon, I noticed that you stepped away from the patient to find the
bag-mask apparatus as the vital signs were deteriorating. I was thinking
there possibly were alternatives means to oxygenate the patient (advocacy).
So I'm curious: how were you seeing the situation at that time? (inquiry)."
Here, the instructor is using advocacy plus inquiry to elicit the invisible
frames that guided the trainee's actions. This is the generic approach that
instructors can use in any scenario: Step (1) notice a relevant result; step
(2) observe what actions seemed to lead to the result; and step (3) use advocacy-inquiry to discover the frames that produced the results.

Compare this utterance with a judgmental version ("Damon, I can't believe it took you 90 seconds to notice that he was desaturating!") or a nonjudgmental "guess what I'm thinking" version ("So, Damon, what was
this patient's saturation when you went to look for the bag-mask apparatus?") The judgmental version, although getting the instructor's point across,
precludes the instructor learning what frames or assumptions set Damon on
a particular path of action; it also may humiliate Damon. The nonjudgmental version leaves Damon uncertain about what the instructor is thinking or
why he is being asked this question; the result will likely be confusion or defensiveness. He may correctly detect that the instructor already knows the
answer to the question and has a judgment that is lurking in the background.
The advocacy-inquiry utterance clearly and directly stated the instructor's
perspective and concerns, and set out to bring to light the meaning-making
process that had Damon focused on finding missing equipment.

The advocacy-inquiry version helps surface Damon's frames. For example, consider the debriefing between Damon and his instructor illustrated in
Box 1. This example, taken from one of the authors' actual debriefings,
shows how advocacy-inquiry spoken with an honest sense of curiosity helps
trainees like Damon learn from simulations by digging deeper into the
frames that drive their actions. It also helps the instructor learn about the
trainees' thought process and provides a lever for deeper teaching. To be
clear, this technique is not about talking nicely. On the contrary, it places
the instructors' thoughts, judgments, and feelings front-and-center. The difference is that by treating the instructor's views as requiring public testing
(by saying their viewpoint in the advocacy and then inviting a different viewpoint with the inquiry), the instructor increases mutuality by opening his or
her own views to challenge and making himself or herself vulnerable to
learning. Additionally, by pairing this advocacy with true inquiry, the instructor increases mutuality by respecting the trainee enough to value his
or her (the trainee's) perspective, and this, in turn, improves learning.

Table 2
Example debriefing dialog to establish individual then group frames

Debriefing Dialog		Commentary
Debriefer	Trainees	
To the group: It looked to me like it was confusing. How did you feel?	Group: Several members agree.	Establish a problematic result (confusion, lack of role clarity).
So, it looked to me as though that confusion may have prevented you from effectively executing respiratory resuscitation and, then, later the ACLS algorithm. How do you all see it?	Group: Yes, the confusion was a problem .	Establish clinical consequences. This shows why lack of role clarity matters.
Diana, it looked to me like you might have been the leader. Did you feel that was your job?	Diana: Yes, I was the leader sort of, but we never said anything about it. And then later, it seemed that Suresh was more in charge.	Explore actions that may have lead to the resulting confusion.
I noticed that too. You looked like you were managing the event, but no one ever said anything.	Diana: Right.	
I was thinking that it would have helped for either you or someone in the group to state explicitly that you were the leader. I am wondering why that did not happen?	Diana: Well, I was not too sure of myself. I mean, the other people are pretty much equal to me and I did not want to seem bossy and unlikable. Also, I was unsure about whether I would do a good job and maybe I would look stupid.	Diana's frame is established (eg, If I am a peer with others it's awkward for me to step up as leader).

Anyone else have a thought?	Eliza: I would have felt much better if I knew Diana was in charge. I certainly did not want to do it and we needed someone to be in charge. But, I did not want to put Diana on the spot.	Beginning to understand Eliza's frame (eg, If asking someone to lead means putting them on the spot, I should not do it).
In my experience, I have occasionally heard someone running an event like this say, "I'll run this event, but you all have to help me." I am curious what you all would have thought if Diana had said something like that?	Ricardo: I would have been relieved and grateful to Diana. Someone has to run it! I guess I could have just confirmed that Diana was the leader.	Group beginning to reframe (eg, Even if I am a bit unsure what to do, it is better to speak up than say nothing).
Turning to Diana: Diana, do you have a thought on this?	Diana: Yes, I can see that is probably a good idea. Then I do not have to look too bossy and I have people on the team who know they have to help me.	Diana moves to a new frame (eg, It is okay to say I want to be the leader if I pair it with a request for help).

The debriefer's goal is that trainees understand the importance of role clarity and establishing an event manager for resuscitations. The example shows how the debriefer (1) helps to identify an important problem (establishing an event manger); (2) uncovers one student's frame; (3) explores other students' frames; (4) facilitates reframing; and (5) offers a new action to deal more effectively with establishing an event manager in the future.

Table 2 provides an example of how to apply the debriefing with good judgment approach. The table shows how the frames-actions-results conceptual model, the instructor's judgments, and advocacy-inquiry fit together to discover the frames that led to a respiratory arrest and chaos in a scenario requiring a cardiac resuscitation.

Summary

The debriefing with good judgment approach is designed to increase the chances that the trainee hears and processes what the instructor is saying without being defensive or trying to guess the instructor's critical judgment. The debriefing with good judgment appellation is not meant to imply that the judgmental or nonjudgmental approach do not have good judgment as their basis. The authors believe that all three approaches often start with some important evaluative insight held by the instructor. We chose the salutary name "debriefing with good judgment" to highlight the positive attributes of the approach. These are, providing trainees with a clear signal about the instructor's point of view while reducing the potential noise (misunderstandings or defensiveness) that too often is associated with the judgmental and nonjudgmental approaches. The judgmental approach poses a substantial risk of embarrassing or humiliating the student and the nonjudgmental approach may send confusing and mixed messages to the learner. Both approaches can obfuscate or reduce the clarity of the instructor's message and the trainee's frames.

The debriefing with good judgment approach has two constraints. The most important is that the model presumes that the trainee is operating with good will and is trying to do the right thing. In those rare cases where the trainee is willfully negligent or malevolent, the model does not work. In those circumstances, other techniques are superior (counseling, goal setting, discipline, and so forth). Second, instructors may find difficulty with this approach when dealing with trainees who come from cultures in which deferring to authority and elders is of paramount importance and inhibits their disclosing views that may seem to contradict those of the instructor. To support the method in this context, explicit preparation regarding the goals and norms of the simulation environment is required, and sometimes even that is not enough.

In debriefing the heat and drama of a high-fidelity clinical simulation, it is easy to focus primarily on trainees' actions. The debriefing with good judgment approach, however, highlights three additional areas of importance. First, it is vital that instructors ask questions like those of an anthropologist, which help bring to the surface and clarify the invisible sense-making process, the cognitive frames, and the emotions that governed the trainee's actions. Second, instructors work to become aware of, and explicitly narrate, their own invisible judgments and concerns about crucial elements of the scenario. But instead of treating their own judgments or concerns as the single truth, they test their views against the trainees' view of the same issue. This does not mean that instructors relinquish their expertise, or disguise their judgments in a sandwich of niceties; rather, they state their view of the situation as a hypothesis and use that as a springboard to legitimize and explore the trainees' view. By understanding how trainees' frames, assumptions, and beliefs drive the actions they take, instructors can match their teaching objectives with problems that are most salient to the trainee. Finally, the debriefing with good judgment approach helps trainees and instructors learn of unintended consequences of common clinical and social frames and assumptions.

Acknowledgment

The authors are grateful to the US Department of Veterans Affairs' Merit Review Entry Program, the Josiah Macy, Jr. Foundation, the Risk Management Foundation of the Harvard Medical Institutions, Richard Nielsen, Boston College, Carroll School of Management, and the Harvard-MIT Division of Health Sciences and Technology for support in developing the ideas and material in this article. They also express thanks to the participants in the Institute for Medical Simulation instructor workshops for giving a forum and their patience to try out and refine these concepts. A version of this article has appeared previously in *Simulation in Healthcare*, under the title "There's no such thing as non-judgmental debriefing: a theory and method for debriefing with good judgment." Simulation in Health Care 2006;1:49–55.

References

[1] Darling M, Parry C, Moore J. Learning in the thick of it. Harv Bus Rev 2005;83(7):84–92.
[2] Dismukes RK, Smith GM. Facilitation and debriefing in aviation training and operations. Aldershot (UK): Ashgate; 2001.
[3] Hankinson H. The cognitive and affective learning effects of debriefing after a simulation game. School of education. Indianapolis (IN): Indiana University; 1987. [116].
[4] Lederman LC. Debriefing: toward a systematic assessment of theory and practice. Simul Gaming 1992;23:145–60.
[5] Morrison JE, Meliza LL. Foundations of the after action review process, Special Report 42. Alexandria (VA): United States Army Research Institute for the Behavioral and Social Science; 1999.
[6] Petranek CF, Corey S, Black R. Three levels of learning in simulations: participating, debriefing, and journal writing. Simul Gaming 1992;23:186–95.
[7] Porter T. Beyond metaphor: applying a new paradigm of change to experiential debriefing. The Journal of Experiential Education 1999;22:85–90.
[8] Steinwachs B. How to facilitate a debriefing. Simul Gaming 1992;23:186–95.
[9] Thiagarajan S. Using games for debriefing. Simul Gaming 1992;23:161–73.
[10] Edmondson A. Psychological safety and learning behavior in work teams. Adm Sci Q 1999; 44:350–83.
[11] Argyris C, Schön DA. Theory in practice: increasing professional effectiveness. Jossey-Bass series in higher education. London: Jossey-Bass; 1974.

[12] Schön D. The reflective practitioner. New York: Basic Books; 1983.
[13] Torbert WR. Learning from experience: toward consciousness. New York: Columbia University Press; 1972.
[14] Senge PM. The fifth discipline: the art and practice of the learning organization. New York: Currency Doubleday; 1990.
[15] Stone D, Patton B, Heen S. Difficult conversations. New York: Penguin Books; 1999.
[16] Rudolph JW, Taylor SS, Foldy EG. Collaborative off-line reflection: a way to develop skill in action science and action inquiry. In: Reason P, Bradbury H, editors. Handbook of action research. Thousand Oaks (CA): Sage; 2001. p. 405–12.
[17] Kegan R, Lahey LL. How the way we talk can change the way we work. San Francisco (CA): Jossey-Bass; 2001.
[18] Friedman VJ. Action science: creating communities of inquiry in communities of practice. In: Reason P, Bradbury H, editors. Handbook of action research: participative inquiry and practice. London: Sage; 2001. p. 159–78.
[19] Schön D. Educating the reflective practitioner: toward a new design for teaching and learning in the professions. San Francisco (CA): Jossey-Bass; 1987.
[20] Argyris C, Schön DA. Organizational learning: a theory of action perspective. Reading (MA): Addison-Wesley; 1978.
[21] Bartunek JM. Changing interpretive schemes and organizational restructuring: the example of a religious order. Adm Sci Q 1984;29:355–72.
[22] Gentner D, Stevens AL. Mental models. Hillsdale (NJ): Lawrence Erlbaum Associates; 1983.
[23] Argyris C, Putnam R, Smith DM. Action science: concepts, methods and skills for research and intervention. San Francisco (CA): Jossey-Bass; 1985.
[24] Steinbruner JD. The cybernetic theory of decision: new dimensions of political analysis. Princeton (NJ): Princeton University Press; 1974.
[25] Watzlawick P, Weakland JH, Fisch R. Change: principles of problem formation and problem resolution. New York: Horton; 1974.
[26] Weick KE. Sensemaking in organizations. Thousand Oaks (CA): Sage; 1995.
[27] Snook SA. Friendly fire: the accidental shootdown of US black hawks over Northern Iraq. Princeton (NJ): Princeton University Press; 2000.
[28] Weick KE, Sutcliffe K, Obstfeld D. Organizing and the process of sensemaking. Organization Science 2005.
[29] Edmondson AE. Learning from mistakes is easier said than done: group and organizational influences on the detection and correction of human error. J Appl Behav Sci 1996;32:5–28.
[30] Scanlon T. What we owe to each other. Cambridge (MA): Belknap Press; 1998.
[31] Leape LL. Error in medicine. JAMA 1994;272:1851–7.
[32] Leape LL. The preventability of medical injury. In: Bogner MS, editor. Human error in medicine. Hillsdale (NJ): Lawrence Erlbaum Associates; 1994. p. 13–25.
[33] Weisinger H. The critical edge: how to criticize up and down your organization and make it pay off. New York: Little Brown and Company; 1989.
[34] Weisinger H. The power of positive criticism. New York: AMACOM; 2000.
[35] Morrison EW, Milliken FJ. Organizational silence: a barrier to change and development in a pluralistic world. Academy of Management Review 2000;25(4):706–25.
[36] Argyris C. Knowledge for action. San Francisco (CA): Jossey-Bass; 1993.
[37] Argyris C. On organizational learning. Cambridge (MA): Blackwell; 1994.

ELSEVIER
SAUNDERS

Anesthesiology Clin
25 (2007) 377–383

ANESTHESIOLOGY
CLINICS

Integration of Standardized Patients into Simulation

Mary J. Cantrell, MA[a,b,]*, Linda A. Deloney, EdD[c]

[a]*Center for Clinical Skills Education and Standardized Patient Program, University of Arkansas for Medical Sciences, 4301 West Markham, #735, Little Rock, AR 72205, USA*
[b]*The PULSE Center, 800 Marshall Street, Slot 852, Little Rock, AR 72202, USA*
[c]*Department of Radiology, College of Medicine, University of Arkansas for Medical Sciences, 4301 West Markham, #556, Little Rock, AR 72205, USA*

The goal of medical education is to prepare physicians to deliver safe, competent, quality patient care. Once in practice, these physicians are expected to integrate their clinical expertise with interpersonal, communication, and professional skills. Their ability to react appropriately to patients' medical problems is derived from knowledge, skills, and attitudes that are acquired over time through training, practice, and repetition.

The confluence of increased clinical workloads, concerns for patient safety, rapid and constant technologic innovations, restrictions on house-staff duty hours, the paradigm shift from apprenticeship to outcomes-based medical education, and the push for maintenance of certification has made physician teaching time much harder to come by in recent years. Medical educators must identify new tools and innovative methods to facilitate teaching and assessment.

One such tool is simulation, a teaching methodology that has experienced rapid growth in medical education. Educational benefits of medical simulation in controlled settings are widely understood. Simulation allows the learner to build knowledge and experience through practice and rehearsal in a safe environment where, fortuitously, the inconvenience, discomfort, and potential harm to "real" patients are minimized. Learners can review and practice procedures as often as they need for mastery.

Effective simulation parallels real world experience in a functional sense, even if it is not realistic in every detail. Simulating the conditions of actual medical practice requires the incorporation of teamwork, leadership, and

---

* Corresponding author.
E-mail address: cantrellmaryj@uams.edu (M.J. Cantrell).

even crisis management. By incorporating aspects of interpersonal and communication skills and medical professionalism (two of the expected competencies for physicians across all educational levels) the conditions become more authentic [1].

A criticism of simulation in the medical environment has been its neglect of the patient as a person. Integrating standardized patient (SP) methodology into high-fidelity simulation increases the potential of the learning experience exponentially. Integrating one or more SPs into a scenario increases the realism, and SP methodology standardizes the simulation, making it reproducible for all learners.

In the health and medical sciences, SPs have been used to provide a safe and supportive environment for learning and assessment for more than 40 years. They do not replace real patients in the medical school curriculum, but rather supplement the learning experience by providing standardized, realistic patient interactions. In the authors' institution, medical students who participated in a comprehensive education program that included one-on-one SP instruction in clinical breast examination were compared with students who received traditional, didactic instruction and practiced on plastic breast models. The students who received standardized training from an SP outscored those who received traditional instruction, not only on a multiple-choice knowledge-base test, but also on the clinical breast examination case in an objective clinical skills examination that was administered at the completion of their physical diagnosis course [2].

Health care encounters rarely happen without a team of nurses, physicians, allied health professionals, or the patient's friends and family in the background. In pharmaceutical education, the SP became "standardized participants" because pharmacists may interact with a patient, physician, or nurse [3]. "Participant" is also more appropriate than "patient" for medical simulation because of the wide variety of roles that may be portrayed during a simulation scenario to increase realism.

There is limited literature about the use of SPs with high-fidelity simulation. This article provides an overview of SP methodology and offers suggestions for integrating SPs into medical simulation scenarios.

Fundamentals of standardized patient methodology

The SP was introduced in 1963 by Barrows [4], a neurologist and junior faculty member at the University of Southern California. Working with Stephen Abrahamson, who was newly recruited to establish one of the first departments of medical education in the United States, Dr. Barrows sought to improve the evaluation of medical students at the conclusion of the neurology clerkship. He challenged himself to develop a case for which he knew every sign and symptom that could be reproduced exactly for every student.

His case came to life as Patty Dugger, a paraplegic woman with multiple sclerosis. A checklist enabled "Patty" to record the details of each encounter as an objective measure of the student's performance. This is the essential SP methodology still used today.

Barrows defined an SP as "a person who has been carefully coached to simulate an actual patient so accurately that the simulation cannot be detected by a skilled clinician." Other terminology has included simulated patient, programmed patient, patient instructor, patient educator, professional patient, surrogate patient, and patient actor. It was Geoffrey Norman, a Canadian psychometrician, who is credited with "standardized patient," the term that is now used routinely throughout medical education. Norman believed "standardized" connoted the idea of making the patient challenge identical for every learner [5].

The SP concept was expanded by Gliva-McConvey [6], who worked with Barrows and one of the first SP trainers in the field, to include "real" patients. She defined an SP as a "person trained to portray a patient scenario, or an actual patient using their own history and physical exam findings, for the instruction, assessment, or practice of communication and/or examining skills of a health care provider." Whether the SP is an able-bodied individual trained to simulate a patient's illness or a patient with stable findings who is trained to present his or her disease, the SP portrays the patient experience in a standardized way.

SPs are medical educator extenders, similar in concept to physician extenders in clinical practice, so they must be selected for their intelligence, dependability, and attention to detail. Some SPs are actors, but others are retirees or homemakers or people with flexible schedules who enjoy altruistic work. Perhaps because the SP methodology originated in "Hollywood," or maybe because actors who have flexible work schedules and are accustomed to accepting part-time, short-term job assignments often work as SPs, there has been a tendency to refer to SPs as "actors" or "actor-patients." Like actors, SPs learn a script and rehearse the role of a character. The character is presented in an educational setting, not a dramatic or theatrical production. Every presentation is standardized, and a guide to every checklist restricts the SP's variation from the script. Another important distinction is that SPs are trained to provide objective reports and subjective ratings of their interactions with the learners. Viewed from a theatrical perspective, then, SPs are the critics, not the performers.

After decades of research demonstrated SP assessment to be valid, reliable, and practical, SP methodology was incorporated into high-stakes testing for medical licensure. In 1993, the Medical Council of Canada became the first entity to use SPs in a licensure examination. The Educational Commission for Foreign Medical Graduates followed by introducing the Clinical Skills Assessment to test the clinical skills of foreign medical graduates in 1998. Then, in 2004, the National Board of Medical Examiners implemented a clinical skills examination using SPs as a component of the United States Medical Licensing Examination.

Advantages and limitations of standardized patients

Multiple applications of SP methodology have been developed in parallel with quality standards for reliability and validity. Advantages of using SPs are shown in Box 1.

SP methodology is limited in that multiple patient encounters may be needed for broad-ranged training or testing. The number of cases a learner sees during an objective structured clinical examination (OSCE), for example, typically ranges from 8 to 12. Another constraint is that SPs may not be able to simulate every physical sign (ie, heart murmurs or lung sounds). Integration with simulation can overcome this limitation.

Integration of standardized patients into simulation

Simulation is a training and feedback method in which learners practice tasks and processes in lifelike circumstances using models or virtual reality. Feedback from observers, peers, or video cameras has been used to assist skills improvement. High-fidelity medical simulation provides a new set of tools for clinical skills development that is similar to professional training

---

Box 1. Advantages of using SPs

Available anytime, any place
Comparable with real patients (valid)
Faculty can control the learning objectives
Faculty can integrate psychosocial issues into a case
Learners can receive immediate and constructive feedback
Learners can practice invasive examinations (pelvic or breast examinations)
Learners can rehearse clinical situations they are not ready to manage alone
Learners performance can be compared
Limits inconvenience, discomfort, or potential harm to real patients
Provides a longitudinal experience in a compressed time frame
Portrayals are standardized and reproducible (reliable)
Reduces time demands on physician teaching faculty
Safe environment minimizes learners anxiety

where there is no zero tolerance for error (aviation, defense, maritime, and nuclear energy).

Adding an SP to the high-fidelity simulation requires some planning and at least a modest budget. If an institution has an SP program, an SP trainer can help develop a simulation plan, hire the SPs, and assist with training and implementation. If an institution does not have an SP program, contact the Association of Standardized Patient Educators to find an experienced trainer in the area.

If one does not have access to a trainer, these few steps enable one to integrate SPs into their simulation. Begin by writing the scenario. Every person in the scenario needs background information to create the level of realism that is required for the high-fidelity simulation. Determine how many SPs would be involved in the scenario. Would a nurse, pharmacist, or an attending physician be in the room? Would the patient be receiving services from an allied health professional, such as a radiology technologist? Might a chaplain or security officer be present? Where are the patient's friends and family members? Rely on experience to create the most realistic scenario possible.

Each SP who participates in the scenario needs a written case statement or script. Give the SP a pseudonym and basic demographic information. Identify the gender, age, and any personal characteristics that describe the SP. Next, describe the relationship of the SP to the simulator. Summarize the medical situation and explain how the simulator came to be in that situation.

Make a checklist of items the SP is to observe during the simulation. Checklist items typically focus on communication and interpersonal skills during a crisis. As a general rule, the checklist should have no fewer than five items and no more than 15. Checklist items might include the following: "The health care worker asked me what happened." "I told the health care worker all the medications my dad is taking." "After I started to cry, a member of the team escorted me out of the ED." Items should be simple, not complex. "The health care worker asked me to tell them where my mother fell and what medicines she takes" is difficult for the SP to score, for example, because it involves more than one action.

After the scenario and cases are written and the simulation is scheduled, contact SPs who fit the descriptions. Those who are interested and can guarantee their availability during the required time frame may be hired as "contract labor" for the simulation. SPs are typically paid by the hour, and should be offered $15 to $20 per hour for a reasonable training period plus the hours spent in the simulation.

After the SP is hired, schedule the first training approximately 2 weeks before the simulation. At the first training, give the SP a brief orientation to the simulator and describe the role the SP will portray. Ask the SP to write down everything said about who the character is and what he or she knows about the patient; this is a good way to reinforce their knowledge of the case. Next, walk the SP through the actions of the encounter. Let the SP feel where he or she will be in the room and where to enter and exit. Allow the SP to walk through each item on the checklist. After this first training, allow the SP a few days to study the material and checklist. After this independent study period, the SP should return to practice the encounter with a group of people who know the case. During this second training, the SP should rehearse and practice a sufficient number of times to ensure accuracy. During this "dry run" the checklist should be used and clarified. If necessary, the checklist can be adjusted by the faculty and finalized for the simulation.

In performing the simulation, the SP presents the medical history, body language, physical findings, and emotional and personality characteristics. The key to interacting with SPs is to relate to them exactly as a real person who has either a professional or personal relationship to the simulator. SPs will not interrupt a learner during an encounter, nor will they volunteer any information. Learners should not attempt to communicate with an SP out of role. This is unprofessional and embarrasses both the SP and the learner.

Feedback and debriefing

After an encounter, SPs can provide immediate and constructive feedback to learners based on their objective reports (checklists) or subjective ratings of interpersonal skills. The debriefing process helps people learn from their experience by reflecting, analyzing, and talking about the experience. It is recommended to debrief the participants immediately after a high-fidelity simulation, while the experience is fresh and it is easy to demonstrate a key point or repeat part of the simulation. A facilitator should guide the process by asking questions, giving feedback, and clarifying information.

Computer simulations with feedback have been shown to be effective and economical supplements to traditional residency training methods. At the University of Washington, clinical anesthesia residents were randomized into simulator-with-debriefing and traditional groups for a 2-year study. The residents in the debriefing group demonstrated improved response to simulated anesthetic emergencies in a mannequin-based anesthesia simulator [7].

Recommended resources

For the medical educator interested in learning more about working with SPs, the following resources are recommended:

- Arizona Clinical Interview Rating Scale. Available at: http://www. spputoronto.ca/docs/ACIR_1_Page_Communication_Skills_scores_blank_ sheet.doc. *Behaviorally anchored checklist to assess medical interviewing skills.*

- Association of Standardized Patient Educators. Available at: http://www.aspeducators.org/. *Link to the international organization for professionals in SP methodology.*
- Barrows HS. Simulated (standardized) patients and other human simulations. Chapel Hill (NC): *Health Sciences Consortium; 1987. Primary guide to the basics of SP training.*
- Barrows HS. Training standardized patients to have physical findings. Southern Illinois University School of Medicine; 1999. *Training guide for presentation of 49 different physical signs by SPs.*
- Phillibert I, editor. ACGME Bulletin, December 2005. Available at http://www.acgme.org/acWebsite/bulletin/bulletin12_05.pdf. *Entire issue devoted to simulation in graduate medical education.*
- Wallace P. Coaching Standardized Patients: for Use in the Assessment of Clinical Competence. New York: Springer Publishing Company; 2006. *Handbook that guides SP trainers in the art of coaching through preparing SPs for portraying patients and the physical examination.*

Summary

SPs can greatly enhance high-fidelity simulation. The educational experience becomes more realistic than by simply using a simulator. If an institution has an SP program, the SP trainer can hire and train SPs for simulation. Once the SPs are trained, the simulation can be replicated many times. The SP's ability to record what happens during the simulation and give feedback to the learner enriches the experience. Faculty are free to participate in the simulation in an observer role, taking notes and concentrating on the learner's performance. The learner's ability to react appropriately to a medical scenario can be assessed by checklists that include ratings of communication and interpersonal skills.

References

[1] Kneebone R, Nestel D, Wetzel C, et al. The human face of simulation: patient-focused simulation training. Acad Med 2006;81(10):919–24.
[2] Heard JK, Cantrell M, Presher L, et al. Using standardized patients to teach breast evaluation to sophomore medical students. J Cancer Educ 1995;10(4):191–4.
[3] Monaghan M, Gardner S, Hastings J, et al. Student attitudes toward the use of standardized patients in a communication course. Am J Pharm Educ 1997;61:131–6.
[4] Barrows HS. An overview of the uses of standardized patients for teaching and evaluating clinical skills. Acad Med 1993;68(6):443–51 [discussion: 451–3].
[5] Wallace P. Following the threads of an innovation: the history of standardized patients in medical education. Caduceus 1997;13(2):5–28.
[6] Gliva-McConvey G, Theresa A. Thomas professional skills center, eastern Virginia medical school; chair, ASPE Standards of Practice Committee. Available at: http://www.aspeducators.org/sp_info.htm. Accessed November 22, 2006.
[7] Schwid HA, Rooke GA, Michalowski P, et al. Screen-based anesthesia simulation with debriefing improves performance in a mannequin-based anesthesia simulator. Teach Learn Med 2001;13(2):92–6.

ELSEVIER
SAUNDERS

Anesthesiology Clin
25 (2007) 385–389

ANESTHESIOLOGY
CLINICS

Index

Note: Page numbers of article titles are in **boldface** type.

A

Academic-private partnership, for statewide simulation systems, 280–281

Adverse event analysis, simulation applications for task performance evaluation, 249–251

American Society of Anesthesiologists (ASA), role in simulation-based teaching and CME, **209–223**
  Committee on simulation education, 216
  Workgroup on simulation education, 213–216

Anesthesia Crisis Resource Management Program, 291

Avatars, in virtual worlds for team training, 327

Aviation, use of simulation in, 306–307

B

Board examinations, in anesthesiology, use of simulation in Israeli, 264–266

Building capacity, models for, in statewide simulation systems, 272–273

C

Capacity, building, models for, in statewide simulation systems, 272–273

Certifying, and credentialing with simulation, **261–269**
  admission to Tel Aviv University Sackler School of Medicine, 263–264
  incorporating into assessment and evaluation, 266–267
  Israeli board examination in anesthesiology, 264–266
  Miller's model of medical competence, 261–262
  objective structured clinical examination, 262–263

Cockpit-crew resource management, use of simulation in, 307–308

Code teams, simulation and improved performance of, 313

Cognition in action, simulation applications for human performance evaluation, 242–244

Competence, Miller's model of medical, 261–262
  simulation in improvement of patient safety and, 230–231

Continuing medical education (CME), in anesthesiology, national program and ASA activities in simulation, **209–223**

Credentialing, and certifying with simulation, **261–269**
  admission to Tel Aviv University Sackler School of Medicine, 263–264
  incorporating into assessment and evaluation, 266–267
  Israeli board examination in anesthesiology, 264–266
  Miller's model of medical competence, 261–262
  objective structured clinical examination, 262–263
  potential of procedural simulation for, 352–353

Crew resource management, team training and, **283–300**
  effectiveness of, 293–296
    didactic classroom-based, 294–295
    simulation *versus* didactic classroom-based, 295–296
    simulation-based, 293–294
  future of, 296
  guidelines for improving patient safety via, 289–290
  principles of, 284–285